CONCISE GUIDE TO

Marriage and Family Therapy

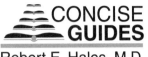

CONCISE
GUIDES

Robert E. Hales, M.D.
Series Editor

CONCISE GUIDE TO
Marriage and Family Therapy

Eva C. Ritvo, M.D.

Associate Professor
Department of Psychiatry and Behavioral Sciences
University of Miami School of Medicine
Chair, Department of Psychiatry and Behavioral Medicine
Mt. Sinai Medical Center
Miami, Florida

Ira D. Glick, M.D.

Professor
Department of Psychiatry
Stanford University School of Medicine
Stanford, California

American Psychiatric Publishing, Inc.

Washington, DC
London, England

This Concise Guide was developed in part from Glick ID, Berman EM, Clarkin JF, Rait DS: *Marital and Family Therapy,* Fourth Edition. Washington, DC, American Psychiatric Press, 2000. Used with permission.

Manufactured in the United States of America on acid-free paper
06 05 04 03 02   5 4 3 2 1
First Edition

American Psychiatric Publishing, Inc.
1400 K Street, N.W.
Washington, DC 20005
www.appi.org

Library of Congress Cataloging-in-Publication Data

Ritvo, Eva C., 1961-
    Concise guide to marriage and family therapy / Eva C. Ritvo, Ira D. Glick. — 1st ed.
        p. ; cm. —(Concise guides series)
    Includes bibliographical references and index.
    ISBN 1-58562-077-7 (alk. paper)
        1. Family psychotherapy. 2. Marital psychotherapy. I. Glick, Ira D., 1935- II. Title. III.
Concise guides (American Psychiatric Publishing)
    [DNLM: 1. Family Therapy—methods. 2. Marital Therapy—methods. WM 430.5.F2
R6156c 2002]
RC488.5.R585 2000
616.89'156—dc21
                                                                                              2002071117

British Library Cataloguing in Publication Data
A CIP record is available from the British Library.

CONTENTS

3 Dysfunctional Families 37

4 Conducting a Family Evaluation 53

5 Formulating an Understanding of the Family Problem Areas 75

---

9 Promoting Change in Family Treatment: Issues of Alliance and Resistance 141

13   Separation and Divorce. 199

14   Indications and Contraindications for
Family Therapy. 215

LIST OF TABLES

LIST OF FIGURES

INTRODUCTION

to the Concise Guides Series

The Concise Guides Series from American Psychiatric Publishing, Inc., provides, in an accessible format, practical information for psychiatrists, psychiatry residents, and medical students working in a variety of treatment settings, such as inpatient psychiatry units, outpatient clinics, consultation-liaison services, and private office settings. The Concise Guides are meant to complement the more detailed information to be found in lengthier psychiatry texts.

The Concise Guides address topics of special concern to psychiatrists in clinical practice. The books in this series contain a detailed table of contents, along with an index, tables, figures, and other charts for easy access. The books are designed to fit into a lab coat pocket or jacket pocket, which makes them a convenient source of information. References have been limited to those most relevant to the material presented.

Robert E. Hales, M.D., M.B.A.
Series Editor, Concise Guides

PREFACE

The path to achieving the knowledge and skills necessary for being a competent family therapist is diverse. Some prefer working with families, that is, with clinical case material, whereas others prefer didactic material. We are strong believers in the notion that students learn in many ways. As such, one of us (I.G.) has recently headed the editorial group that revised and updated the fourth edition of our text on marital and family therapy.[1]

This Concise Guide is a direct descendant of that work. It is written for those who asked us to succinctly encapsulate the core material needed by a student (or a seasoned practitioner) in the diverse settings of current family treatment practice around the world.

Thus, this guide describes the basics of marital and family therapy. The teaching plan can be clearly seen in the table of contents. A moment's study here will greatly reward the student in the long run. In Chapter 1, we provide a brief background and introduction of terms. Next, in Chapter 2, we set the stage for treatment by describing what functional families look like. In Chapter 3, we focus on problems and dysfunction from a family systems prospective. Once that material is understood, in Chapter 4 the issue is to coherently organize the material, that is, to do an evaluation and a genogram. In Chapter 5, we describe what is crucial to the entire process—making a diagnosis of the family (and its individuals) and

---

[1]Glick ID, Berman E, Clarkin JF, et al: *Marital and Family Therapy,* 4th Edition. Washington, DC, American Psychiatric Press, 2000.

establishing a treatment "contract" (meaning, "How are we going to work together to change this situation?").

Now we are ready in Chapter 6 to discuss therapy, the first step of which is determining goals. In Chapter 7, we describe our integrated model, the basic strategies of family intervention, and techniques for reorganizing the family structure. In Chapter 8, for heuristic reasons, we dissect the phases of the course of treatment. In Chapter 9, we address how to build an alliance and deal with the forces working against change. In Chapter 10, we pull together the essential issues involved in conducting the treatment—logistics, setting fees, and, increasingly importantly, combining it with other treatments like medication and individual intervention.

In Chapters 11 and 12, we discuss the issues that are unique to understanding and treating a couple, including evaluation and treatment of sexual dysfunction. In Chapter 13, we focus on the process and management of separation and divorce.

In Chapter 14, we describe the complex issues of when to recommend family therapy and when its use would be inappropriate. Chapter 15 closes this volume with the pearls involved in the ethical and professional issues that are inherent in marital and family treatment.

For a fuller elaboration of all of these topics, we recommend supplementation with the text cited in this preface or specialized journal articles. When in doubt, trust the scientific data that exist— but also value your instincts. The aim of family therapists is to improve the lives of the couples and the families whom we serve.

DEVELOPMENT OF THE FIELD AND DEFINITIONS

■ DEFINITION OF MARRIAGE AND FAMILY THERAPY

Family therapy is distinguished from other psychotherapies by its conceptual focus on the family system as a whole. In this view, major emphasis is placed on understanding how the system as a whole remains functional and on understanding individual behavior patterns as arising from, and inevitably feeding back into, the complex interactions within the family system. In other words, a person's thoughts, feelings, and behaviors are seen as multidetermined and partly a product of significant interpersonal relationships. From the family systems perspective, alterations in the larger marital and family unit may therefore have positive consequences for the individual members as well as for the larger system. A major emphasis is generally placed on understanding and intervening in the family system's current patterns of interaction, with usually only a secondary interest in the origins and development of these interactions (depending on the model).

Marital and family treatment can be defined as a systematic effort to produce beneficial changes in a marital or family unit by introducing changes into the pattern of family interactions. Its aim is the establishment of more satisfying ways of living for the entire family and for individual family members.

A continuum exists between the intrapsychic system, the interactional family system, and the sociocultural system. Different conceptual frameworks are used when dealing with these systems. A therapist may choose to emphasize any of the points on this continuum, but the family therapist is especially sensitive to and trained in those aspects that relate specifically to the family system—to both its individual characteristics and the larger social matrix.

Although many clinicians agree that problematic interaction may occur in families containing an individual with gross disturbance, it is not always clear whether the faulty interaction is the cause or the effect of the behavior of the disturbed individual. Some practitioners continue to perceive and treat the disequilibrium in the intrapsychic organization of the individual as the central issue, viewing the contextual social matrix of development and adaptation (and most particularly the family) as adding an important dimension to their conceptualization and treatment. Others see and treat as the central issue the disequilibrium in the family, viewing the individual symptoms as the result of, or the attempted solution to, a family problem (Committee on the Family 1970; Minuchin 1974).

For the present, there is reason to believe that both views are important. Pending further research and experience in this area, it seems prudent for the clinician to evaluate each clinical situation carefully, attempting both to understand the phenomena and to select intervention strategies designed to achieve the desired ends.

■ CORE CONCEPTS

General Systems Theory

Family therapy is based on a theory that was developed in the 1970s and that combines a general systems view of interactions, a cybernetic epistemology, traces of interpersonal psychiatry, and the most recent contributions of social constructivism. Thus, we begin this section with a delineation of the basic concepts underlying recent developments in understanding family process and family intervention. These concepts are not numerous, but their paucity belies the profound shift in focus that occurs when one progresses from concepts about the individual to a description of a system and its functioning.

The biologist Von Bertalanffy is credited as being the first to introduce principles that provide an organismic approach to understanding biological beings. He gave these concepts the title *general systems theory* (Von Bertalanffy 1968). Von Bertalanffy believed that the reductionistic, mechanistic tradition in science was insufficient to explain the behavior of living organisms, because this approach depended on a linear series of stepwise cause-and-effect equations. In contrast to this view, Von Bertalanffy developed general principles, which he used to explain biological processes that include considerable complexity and levels of organization. A systems approach emphasizes the relationship between the parts of a complex whole and the context in which these events occur, rather than an isolation of events from their context (Anonymous 1972).

To regulate its exchange with systems outside of itself, the living system must have boundaries (Figures 1–1 and 1–2). The organized family system has a boundary between itself and the surrounding neighborhood and community. This boundary consists of the implicit or explicit rules by which the family keeps information and activities to itself or allows outside information and contact with people in the neighborhood and the community. A family must have clear boundaries in order to be functional. The same is true for subsystems within the family. For example, for the marital subsystem to function, it must have a boundary that separates it from other subsystems, such as the sibling subsystem.

Minuchin (1974) described families as existing on a continuum, from disengaged (i.e., having inappropriately rigid boundaries) to enmeshed (i.e., having overly permeable, diffuse boundaries). Families in the middle of the continuum (having clear boundaries) are considered to be the most functional.

Cultural variations must be taken into account. For example, in some groups, such as upper-class English families, it is customary to send children to boarding school by age 9 or 10, whereas in Hispanic and other cultures, children live at home until they are in their twenties or are married.

Recognition of the existence of subsystems within the family system relates to another notion about organization, *hierarchical*

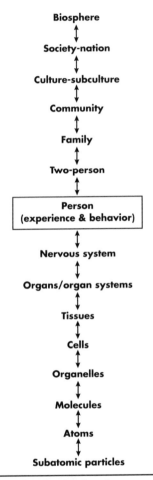

FIGURE 1–1. **Hierarchy of natural systems.**

Source. Reprinted from Engel G: "The Clinical Application of the Biopsycho-social Model." *American Journal of Psychiatry* 137:535–544, 1980. Copyright 1980, American Psychiatric Association. Used with permission.

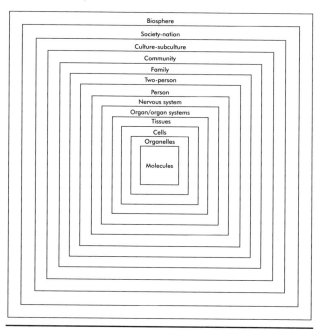

FIGURE 1–2. **Continuum of natural systems.**

Source. Reprinted from Engel G: "The Clinical Application of the Biopsychosocial Model." *American Journal of Psychiatry* 137:535–544, 1980. Copyright 1980, American Psychiatric Association. Used with permission.

organization. The system itself is organized on one or many hierarchical levels entailing systems or subsystems (see Figures 1–1 and 1–2).

In addition to organization, a functional living system must have some means of controlled adaptation to its environment. In 1948, Wiener introduced the notion of cybernetics as a branch of science dealing with control mechanisms and the transmission of information. Wiener pointed out the similarities between the mechanisms of internal control and communication in an animal and in machines. A key concept in cybernetics is that of feedback and the feedback loop.

In this circular sequence of events, element A influences element B, which influences element C, which in turn influences element A. Such mechanisms serve to control the state of the organism or environment (Wiener 1948). These control concepts, such as homeostasis and feedback, have been used by family theorists to understand and change family systems (Jackson 1957; Minuchin et al. 1975).

A third key concept relevant to living systems is that of energy and information. Living systems are open systems, in which energy can be transported in and out of the system. Instead of a tendency toward entropy and degradation of energy, which occurs in nonliving systems, living systems have a tendency toward increased patterning, complexity, and organization. In human open systems such as the family, information (i.e., knowledge from outside of the family) acts as a type of energy that informs the system and can lead to more complex interaction.

To summarize, the family systems approach is a theoretical framework commonly used by family therapists. The understanding of families is ecological in that the capabilities of the family are viewed as greater than the sum of its parts. Each person is viewed in interactive relations with the other family members, all of whom function to maintain the family system coherently but each of whom also strives for his or her own unique goals. A key concept here is that, despite the fact that to an outside observer some behavior appears crazy or self-defeating, this is assumed to be the family's best solution to their problems.

Classical family therapy examines interpersonal relationships—rather than biological, intrapsychic, or societal processes—in attempting to understand human distress. This is not to say that family therapy ignores the intrapsychic or the biological, but its primary vision and interventions are focused on interpersonal relationships.

Family Systems Theory and Homeostasis Over Time

Indeed, it can be said that the critical issue for families is which homeostasis to evolve toward—what to preserve of the past (to manage the present competently) and what to look forward to in the future. Hoffman (1983) developed a useful diagram (Figure 1–3),

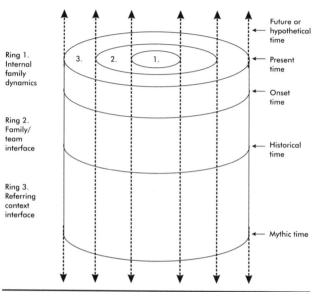

FIGURE 1–3. **Hoffman's time capsule.**

Source. Hoffman L: "A Co-evolutionary Framework for Systemic Family Therapy," in *Diagnosis and Assessment in Family Therapy, The Family Therapy Collections.* Edited by Hansen JC, Keeney BP. Rockville, MD, Aspen Publications, 1983, p. 42.

which she called a time capsule, to illustrate 1) how the family (and treating team) interface with the community and with its internal dynamics and 2) that each family has a long history ("mythic time") and is constantly evolving.

An Integrative Interpersonal Model

Throughout this edition, we base our update of this model on the work of J. M. Lewis (1998) in interpersonal relationships and individual outcome. Our model is based on the notion that there is an ongoing interplay between psychopathology (related to both biological as well as developmental factors) and individual relationships with significant others. As Lewis (1998) has noted,

> At its center this perspective holds that relational structures—the more or less enduring patterns of interaction—either facilitate or impede the continued maturation of the participants. It is important to note that the relationship between an individual and his or her relational system is not linear; rather, individual characteristics influence system properties, and these properties shape individual characteristics.

■ DIFFERENTIATION OF FAMILY THERAPY FROM OTHER PSYCHOTHERAPIES

Family therapy as a format of treatment can be distinguished from other psychotherapies by a fundamental paradigm shift that assumes that people are best understood as operating in systems and that treatment must include all relevant parts of the system. From this come different goals, focuses, participants, and so forth (Table 1–1).

The strategies and techniques of family therapy, whether structural, strategic, multigenerational, behavioral, psychoeducational, experiential, supportive, or psychodynamic, overlap with these same techniques as they are used in individual and group formats. They may, however, take on added dimensions in a family session.

The model of psychopathology underlying family treatment is quite different from other forms of intervention. The family model is based on the assumption that personality development, symptom formation, and therapeutic change result, at least in part, from the family's function as an interdependent transactional unit.

Modern biopsychiatry is concerned with the biological correlates of emotional disorders, whereas personality psychology and the psychotherapies are concerned with individual psychodynamics and their relation to mental disorders. Family therapy is primarily concerned with the relationships among persons and how these family relationships and disruptions are linked both to physical and mental disorders of individuals and to larger contexts in the community.

TABLE 1–1. Family therapy format compared with other psychosocial therapy formats

Therapy format	Intermediate goals	Final goals	Focus	Participants	Length or frequency of sessions	Mean overall duration of treatment
Family	Improve family communication; decrease family conflict	Improved family functioning	Family intervention: family coalitions and roles	Nuclear family unit; extended family; 1–2 therapists	Most 1–2 hours per week	2 months–2 years
Individual	Insight into intrapsychic conflicts; insight into interaction (transference)	Individual personality/ symptom change	Unconscious conflicts; individual's thoughts, wishes, and behaviors	1 patient; 1 therapist	1 hour, 1–5 times per week	2 months–5 years
Group	Sharing with group; improved relating skills in group	Improved individual social functioning	Group participants and feedback	6–8 patients; 1–2 therapists	1.5 hours, 1 time per week	6 months–2 years

Source. Reprinted from Glick ID, Berman EM, Clarkin JF, et al: *Marital and Family Therapy,* 4th Edition. Washington, DC, American Psychiatric Press, 2000, p. 63. Copyright 2000, American Psychiatric Press, Inc. Used with permission.

■ REFERENCES

Anonymous: Towards the differentiation of a self in one's own family, in Family Interaction: A Dialogue Between Family Researchers and Family Therapists. Edited by Framo JL. New York, Springer, 1972, pp 111–166

Committee on the Family: Field of Family Therapy, Report No. 78. New York, Group for the Advancement of Psychiatry, 1970, p 534

Hoffman L: A co-evolutionary framework for systemic family therapy, in Diagnosis and Assessment in Family Therapy, The Family Therapy Collections. Edited by Hansen JC, Keeney BP. Rockville, MD, Aspen Publications, 1983, p 42

Jackson DD: The question of family homeostasis. Psychiatr Q Suppl 31:79–90, 1957

Lewis JM: For better or worse: interpersonal relationships and individual outcome. Am J Psychiatry 155:582–589, 1998

Minuchin S: Families and Family Therapy. Cambridge, MA, Harvard University Press, 1974

Minuchin S, Baker L, Rosman B, et al: A conceptual model of psychosomatic illness in children. Arch Gen Psychiatry 32:1031–1038, 1975

Von Bertalanffy L: General Systems Theory. New York, George Braziller, 1968

Wiener N: Cybernetics, or Control and Communication in the Animal and the Machine. Cambridge, MA, MIT Press, 1948

2

THE FUNCTIONAL FAMILY

There is probably little need to stress the general importance of marriage and the family. These social institutions have existed throughout recorded history in all places and at all times. Even now, despite the talk in some quarters about the death of the family, family and marital relationships, although changing, are clearly very much with us.

However, expectations regarding marriage and the family have changed, especially when we compare the traditional American family with radical modifications of this pattern. The variety of accepted patterns (including cohabitation, stepfamilies, single-parent families, and two- and three-generation families) for marriage and the family is a cause for uncertainty, instability, and distress. Nevertheless, this diversity offers a richness of solutions that a more rigid pattern could not. Anyone engaging in family or couples therapy must be cautioned against thinking of families in any single way.

■ THE FAMILY AS A SYSTEM

Marriages and families differ from other human groups in many ways, including the duration, intensity, and function of their relationships. For human beings, the family constitutes the most important group in relation to individual psychological development, emotional interaction, and maintenance of self-esteem. For many of us, the family is a group in which we experience our strongest loves and hates and in which we enjoy our deepest satisfactions and suffer our most painful disappointments. The characteristics of a family (or of a marriage) as a unit are different from the mere sum of its components.

Family members are usually bound together by intense and long-lasting ties of past experiences, social roles, mutual support and needs, and expectations. Factors are constantly at work to keep the family system in equilibrium and to keep it from undergoing too severe or rapid change.

Family homeostasis refers to the concept that the family is a system designed to maintain a relatively stable state so that, when the whole system or any part of it is subjected to a disequilibrating force, feedback will restore the preexisting equilibrium. However, it is often necessary for the family to move to a new equilibrium. This happens at transition points in the family's life cycle or after a major life change (e.g., a mother goes back to work) or trauma (e.g., an automobile accident in which a family member is injured and cannot continue usual roles).

For the system to be functional, it must have certain characteristics. Table 2–1 presents the 10 processes that characterize functional—that is, healthy or normal—families (Walsh 1993).

■ THE MARITAL/FAMILY LIFE CYCLE

Because one central function of the family is to raise children to adulthood, the system needs to ensure that various phase-specific psychosocial tasks are mastered at each stage of the family life cycle. Stressors during any of these stages may interfere with the accomplishment of normal developmental tasks. Although the family's ability to pass successfully from one specific developmental phase to another may depend on how prior stages have been negotiated, families sometimes find themselves better suited to meet the challenges of one stage than of another.

Couples' ability to communicate clearly, to solve problems, and to maintain a relationship that is reasonably free of projection and incompatible agendas is based on the intrapsychic needs of the individuals, the reflexive behaviors they bring from their families of origin, the evolving marital dynamics, and the state of marital

---

TABLE 2–1. **Processes that characterize functional families**

---

1. Connectedness and commitment of members as a caring, mutually supportive unit
2. Respect for individual differences and autonomy, fostering the development and well-being of members of each generation, from youngest to eldest
3. For couples, a relationship characterized by mutual respect, support, and equitable sharing of power and responsibilities
4. For nurturance, protection, and socialization of children and caregiving to other vulnerable family members, effective parental/executive leadership and authority
5. Organizational stability, characterized by clarity, consistency, and predictability in patterns of interaction
6. Adaptability: flexibility to meet internal or external demands for change, to cope effectively with stress and problems, and to master normative and nonnormative challenges and transitions across the life cycle
7. Open communication characterized by clarity of rules and expectations, pleasurable interaction, and a range of emotional expression and empathic responsiveness
8. Effective problem-solving and conflict-resolution processes
9. A shared belief system that enables mutual trust, problem mastery, connectedness with past and future generations, ethical values, and concern for the larger human community
10. Adequate resources for basic economic security and psychosocial support in extended kin and friendship networks and community and larger social systems

---

development. Certain normative patterns of stress are determined by the individual and family life cycles, as described in the following paragraphs (Table 2–2).

The Individual Life Cycle

Issues of marriage and family life are greatly affected by the age of the adult participants. Adult developmental phases can be roughly divided into early adulthood, ages 20–40; middle adulthood, ages 40–65; and older adulthood, ages 65 and over.

TABLE 2–2. **The family life cycle and adult development**

Early adulthood (age 20–40 years)

Age 20–30 years
1. Establish an independent life structure—home, friends, etc.
2. Renegotiate relationships with parents
3. Make first set of decisions around occupational choice
4. Explore intimacy/sexuality
5. Possibly deal with parenthood

Age 30 transition
Sometimes rethink early choices—"course correction"

Age 30–40 years
1. Settle into chosen life structure
2. Deepen commitment to work and intimate relationships
3. Experience self as fully adult

Mid-adulthood (age 40–60 years)

Age 40–50 years
1. Deal with complexities of being command generation: may be responsible for children and/or aging parents
2. Midlife transition: reevaluate life goals, work, and relationships
3. Forgive self for sins of omission and commission

Age 50–60 years
1. Settle into life one chose in 40s
2. Accept who one has become
3. Deal with grandparenthood
4. Deal with issues of aging and mortality

Older adulthood (age 60+ years)

Age 60+ years
1. Conduct a life review
2. Give up being command generation
3. Find function and direction in a world that values youth
4. Deal with physical changes of aging

Age 75+ years
Focus on functioning despite physical aging

Source.   Reprinted from Glick ID, Berman EM, Clarkin JF, et al: *Marital and Family Therapy,* 4th Edition, 2000, p. 63. Copyright 2000, American Psychiatric Press, Inc. Used with permission.

Developmental issues in early adulthood include launching from one's family of origin and developing a sense of identity and life structure, a job or career track, and an intimate and committed relationship. In the twenties, when there is a need to attend to all developmental tasks at once, both marital choice and couple development can be profoundly altered by a person's relationship with parents and work. Early love relationships in particular can develop in response to perceived parental demands, a wish to prove oneself as an adult, or a need for a partner to combat fears of being alone. In the twenties, much time and emotional energy may be channeled into work rather than relationships. However, the need to establish the security of emotional ties is great, and most people develop intense, long-term relationships by the late twenties and want to establish a family soon afterward. If they are pleased with their choices, the thirties can be a particularly stable and settled time.

Midlife issues are complex. The early forties are not always a crisis period but are usually characterized by a sense of transition and a need to reevaluate one's life structure after 20 years of functioning adulthood. A sense of mortality and of advancing age prompts many people to review their lives and to redirect some portions of their lives. As spouses, people in midlife may be more willing to forgo an obsession with work and to become more intimate or to forgo a focus on the family and to become more world oriented. Some persons become dissatisfied with their marriages as part of their life review and have extramarital relationships, separations, or divorces. Later midlife can be a source of satisfaction, when people come to terms with who they are and are not. If the marriage is good, it can be a particular source of comfort and strength at this time.

The tasks of older adulthood are to develop a sense of purpose for the rest of life and to review one's life. Because many older adults today can expect to live into their eighties and nineties, the task of finding a purpose and a function in a society that values youth and denigrates age is a difficult one. Questions about how much to rely on adult children and how to construct a meaningful life are key. Because women live an average of 7 years longer than

men and tend to marry men older than themselves, the older population consists primarily of widowed and divorced women, who are
subject to sexism, ageism, and poverty.

Phase of Relationship and Task

In this section on the family life cycle, we first discuss the tasks involved in the beginning family and then those concerning the adult
life cycle as they relate to the family form.

Courtship and Early Marriage

For many people, the most important decision made in the course
of a lifetime is whom they marry. Couple formation is best done
when one has completed the tasks of restructuring one's relationship with one's parents, learned enough about oneself to be aware
of one's characteristic problems, and experienced enough freedom
and adventure that the demands of an intense relationship feel comforting rather than constricting. A new couple preparing for marriage must establish a couple identity, develop effective ways of
communicating and solving problems, and begin to establish a mutual pattern of relating to parents, friends, and co-workers. Decisions about sexuality and some pattern of sexual relating commonly
occur before marriage.

If a couple has not had an intimate sexual relationship before
marriage, sexuality and mutuality will be dealt with in the early
months of the marriage. Ways of communicating and dividing tasks
set up in the first months are often difficult to alter later on, so it is
critical to address these directly and early.

Marriage between people under age 21 often represents a
search for a substitute parent, a way of getting out of a troubled
home or of getting revenge on a parent, or a search for security.
Some of these early marriages function well and allow the partners
to grow, but many interfere with further individuation, especially if
children are born very soon afterward.

Marriages undertaken during the usual time span, from age 21
to the early thirties, are embedded in the set of multiple, complex

tasks of early adulthood. Early marriages are hectic because of the multiple tasks required of young adults. Competency in intimate life, work life, and parenting all must be developed simultaneously. Common stress points in early adult marriage are 1) the birth of children, 2) attempting an egalitarian marriage in a nonegalitarian culture, 3) major transitions in work responsibilities, and 4) illness in a family member.

Marriages between midlife people differ depending on whether they are long-term first marriages or new marriages. Long-term marriages are often threatened by the stirrings of midlife transition, the launching of children, and the beginning of illness. As a result of these types of adversity, these marriages may grow stronger and deeper; but if they are only structural shells, they are likely to suffer. New marriages in midlife are usually second marriages and may benefit from the mistakes of the past. Both members may be more relaxed about themselves and their work and more available for family life. Therefore, the children of second marriages may be easier to raise. However, stepfamily issues may greatly complicate second marriages.

Like marriages in midlife, those between older people may be relationships of habit and convenience or may be deeply connected. In later life, spouses have usually stopped trying to change each other and may be more accepting. However, the rate of divorce has risen even in this age group in recent years. In many marriages in later life, the husband's retirement may put stress on the marriage, but health and illness are the biggest determinants of couple functioning in later years.

Marital Coalition

The core of the family is the *marital coalition*, that is, the couple working together. This term implies that the spouses have been able to loosen their ties appropriately from their families of origin and have been able to develop a sense of their own individuality and self-worth as well as an identity as a couple. Marriage is not merely a joining together of two individuals; it is also a distillation of their families of origin, each with its own experiences, history, lifestyle, and attitudes. One marries not only an individual, but the individual's family of origin as well. Even when the extended family is not physically present, the patterns experienced by the spouses in their original families inevitably influence their current marital and family interactions.

The process of working out a satisfactory marital relationship requires shared agreements between the two people involved. These agreements may consist of explicit rules, implied rules (to which the couple would agree if they were aware of them), and rules that an observer would note but that the couple itself would probably deny. The central or basic rules for interpersonal relationships exist in the five dimensions shown in Table 2–3, which determine the quality of a relationship (Lewis 1998).

TABLE 2–3. **Dimensions of a relationship**

---

1. *Power:* Who is in charge? This is a complex area because there are many kinds of power, ranging from expertise to physical coercion to custom. Although power may be shared in many ways, there is general agreement in most couples about who is in charge if a joint decision is impossible, and whose needs come first in the family.

2. *Closeness-distance:* Partners negotiate what type of emotional distance feels close and intimate and what feels too distant.

3. *Separateness and intimacy—that is, inclusion and exclusion:* Who else is considered to be part of the marital system? This question of boundaries applies not only to actual relatives and other persons, but also to time allocated for career and recreational interests.

4. *Marital commitment:* Both partners need to feel that both they and their spouse are committed to the relationship and are primary in each other's lives.

5. *Intimacy, i.e., the reciprocal sharing of vulnerabilities:* Partners often vary in their need for verbal sharing, but for most couples, this is an important or essential part of bonding.

Couples matched for variables of socioeconomic class; religious, ethnic, and racial backgrounds; and political and social attitudes and values tend to be more successful than less well matched couples. However, dissimilarity or complementarity of personality styles may actually enhance a partnership, as may other subsidiary interests. The determining factor seems to be a match of roles to goals, that is, to achieve a specific goal, whether one needs to choose a partner who is the same as or different from oneself. Temperament and personality factors are another set of key determinants. Two recent studies (Markman, as quoted in Talan 1988; Thomas and Olson 1993) discuss the best predictors of a good marriage. Markman, quoted in Talan (1988), suggests that they "include communication, the ability to resolve conflict, personality compatibility, realistic expectations, and agreement on religious values." What is common in both studies is the ability for couples to resolve differences and communicate differing needs. In our experience, marriages that seem most stable over time are those in which each partner is willing to be influenced by the other and to share power. Predictors of divorce include "stonewalling, criticism, defensiveness, and contempt for the spouse" (Gottman and Levenson 1999).

The Family Life Cycle in Relation to Parents and Children

Although stability and homeostasis are important elements of marital and family systems, inevitably there are other forces that are continually changing the family, pushing it in the direction of development and differentiation. Some of these forces constitute the growth pattern known as the family life cycle. The family life cycle can be thought of as the expected life events that most families go through in a fairly predictable, but not unvarying, sequence. Other stresses can be thought of as unexpected in that they are extraordinary; most families do not necessarily experience them or they occur outside the normal sequence of the life cycle.

The longitudinal view (what we are referring to as the traditional view of the family's development) is analogous to the individual's life cycle (Duvall 1967). As in individual development, the family evolves through expected phases. Table 2–4 shows the traditional phases. Figure 2–1 shows the family life cycle and the approximate years associated with each phase (Duvall 1967).

Children and Shifts in Function

If one imagines that a different family structure develops at each developmental stage, one can also see how most families fundamentally alter their organization in order to change. For example, the marital couple's organization alters dramatically with the birth of the first child, and the structure of this threesome necessarily shifts with the birth of a second child.

The family with young children is characterized by closeness, bonding, and intense inward focus on the infants or young children. In acquiring the role of parents, the married couple faces new responsibilities. Parents must develop and revise strategies for meeting their own needs as well as their child's emerging requirements (Feldstein and Rait 1990). The couple must learn to operate in a triangular situation and to negotiate around what are often different styles of child rearing. Most often the mother is the one who provides most of the child care and cuts back on her professional work, leaving the couple to find a way to negotiate new roles.

TABLE 2–4. **Traditional phases of family development**

Couple formation (love, cohabitation or engagement, marriage)

The childbearing family (birth of the first child, oldest child under 5 years old)

The family with schoolchildren

The family with teenagers

The family as a launching center (the offspring begin their own adult life structure, usually but not always moving away from home)

The family in its middle years (which may include one or both spouse's retirement and often includes grandparenthood)

The couple as part of a three-generation family (includes eventual death of a spouse)

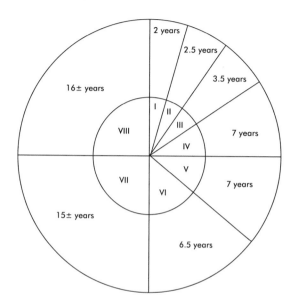

Phase	Family phase	Family description
I	Beginning family	Married couple without children
II	Childbearing family	Oldest child up to age 30 months
III	Family of preschool children	Oldest child age 30 months to 6 years
IV	Family of schoolchildren	Oldest child age 6–13 years
V	Family with teenagers	Oldest child age 13–20 years
VI	Family as launching center	First child gone to last child leaving home
VII	Family in the middle years	Empty nest to retirement
VIII	Aging family	Retirement to death of both spouses

FIGURE 2–1. **The family life cycle.**

Source. Reprinted from Glick ID, Berman EM, Clarkin JF, et al: *Marital and Family Therapy,* 4th Edition. Washington, DC, American Psychiatric Press, 2000, p. 71. Copyright 2000, American Psychiatric Press, Inc. Used with permission.

The family with school-age children is opened up to extrafamilial sources such as the school, families of children's friends, and new peers. As children interact with others outside the family, parents are freed to pursue their own interests. This is a time when children and parents can become good companions and is often a warm and easy time for the family. Even grandparents contribute to the opening up of the family system by introducing their grandchildren to experiences in different contexts. Issues of discipline, values, and amount of freedom for growing children may become major areas of argument. Religious or cultural differences between the parents must be negotiated (around the child) because this issue directly affects the family's rituals and functioning.

As children become adolescents, they press for greater autonomy. At the same time, parents begin to struggle with contradictory desires for family closeness and freedom. The years of adolescence are often difficult for many families. For the first time, the teenager appears to be half in and half out of the family. To manage the developmental tasks of this phase, the family must be strong, flexible, and able to support growth. For most families, however, adolescence is not a time of chaos and rebellion. Parents and children still connect and learn from each other in powerful ways during this time. At the same time, many parents also contend with changes in their own parents' health, leaving them feeling sandwiched between the needs of their children and those of their own parents.

If the adolescent stage involves expected conflicts about how much to hold on and how much to let go, the family with grown children contends with loss as it encourages the achievement of independence and new attachments. The primary task of the family is to continue the letting-go process that began in adolescence, which involves restructuring the relationship while continuing to be related.

■ FAMILY TASKS

Families can be viewed as laboratories for the social, psychological, and biological development and maintenance of family members. In providing this function, couples and families must accomplish vital tasks, including the provision of basic physical needs (food, shelter, and clothing), the development of a marital coalition and the socialization of children, and the resolution of crises that can arise in relation to illness and other life changes.

Provision of Basic Physical Needs

Therapists working with economically disadvantaged families immediately recognize the fundamental requirement of addressing the basic physical and material needs of families. All of the more complex functions of the family are affected by the extent to which these needs are met.

Rearing and Socialization of Children

For the purposes of this discussion, we define *personality* as each person's adaptation to the biological characteristics that he or she inherits at birth and that interact with the demands of the family and the external world. Although much of children's essential temperaments are inborn, their ultimate stance in relation to the world, their knowledge of cultural norms, and their attitudes toward men and women are developed within the family and the neighborhood, as well as through the media (especially television). Early neglect, trauma, or chaotic upbringing can permanently damage brain structure and function.

Children learn from who their parents are as well as from what they do. For this reason, some aspects of learning cannot be controlled by education. An anxious parent will communicate some anxiety to the child, regardless of the parent's skill in communicating. However, we know that certain basic parenting skills are necessary for optimal child development.

Use of Age-Appropriate Child-Rearing Techniques

Parents need to understand the child's capacities at different ages in order to parent adequately. For example, expecting a 1-year-old to demonstrate patience and self-control or trying to reason with a 3-year-old having a temper tantrum will result in rage and confusion for both the child and the parent. In addition, some parents may have particular difficulty with a certain phase because of what they experienced in their own families of origin. For example, a parent who was very sexually promiscuous as an adolescent may become frightened when his or her child reaches the same age and may be untrusting and overly controlling.

Maintenance of Parental Coalition and Generational Boundaries

It is beneficial for both parents and children for the parents to be clear that they are functioning as a team to parent the children and that adult roles are different from child roles. Although parents cannot agree on everything, there should be some sort of mutual, consistent child-rearing guidelines. Even when parents disagree, the child should know that the parents will find a way to deal with the disagreement rather than leave the child in limbo. Problems arise when the parents are so much in conflict that one or both turn to the child for support, leaving the child either with a loyalty conflict ("If I side with Dad, Mom will not love me") or in a "parentified," caregiving role.

Support of a Sibling Coalition

The history of developmental theory has largely neglected the roles of siblings in families. A key issue concerns the microenvironment of the siblings, or the world of the siblings as opposed to that of their parents. Research in the 1990s (Reiss et al. 1991) found that siblings display a small degree of similarity in personality, but this appears to result mostly from shared genes rather than from shared experience. There are obviously other factors that go into how siblings turn out differently—the so-called nonshared environment—such as life events, each child's perceptions about parents, different attitudes of parents to different siblings, and the friends that they develop (Reiss et al. 1991). Family theory has stressed the important role that siblings play in normal family functioning. Each sibling has a crucial role in the maintenance of homeostasis for that particular family system. Siblings often work together when their parents are continually at odds or have divorced or when one or both parents have severe mental illness. That bond is often the link to keep a family functional when one or both parents cannot carry out parental roles.

Family therapists believe that issues of loyalty, attachment, and bonding are important and useful in changing dysfunctional patterns. Dysfunctional families often have dysfunctional sibling relationships. For example, siblings may mimic the parental relationship by always bickering in the same way in which the parents bicker or by one sibling's being dominant. The bottom line for the family therapist is that each sibling should be seen as a separate individual.

Interventions focused on siblings may be included in family treatment models. Treatment can use older siblings as change agents, or focus on sibling conflict. When one parent has died, siblings are important in maintaining the family system in coping with the parental loss. When one sibling has a mental disorder, the others can be active sources of support. In addition, siblings need to know very specific information about Axis I disorders, such as schizophrenia, particularly its prognosis and the resultant difficulties in communication and problem solving with their siblings (Landeen et al. 1992).

■ ALTERNATIVE FAMILY FORMS

Family forms that result from shifts in companionship status are 1) cohabitation and serial relationships, 2) the family during separation and divorce, 3) binuclear and single-parent families, and 4) remarried families or stepfamilies. As the life cycle lengthens and people can expect 50, 60, or even 70 years of functional adulthood, the possibility that one will have only one partner, chosen in one's early twenties, for all of one's life seems more remote than ever.

Serial Relationships

Some people develop a life pattern of sequential relationships, which includes several long-term serious relationships and may include several marriages with the creation and dissolution of two or three family units. It is often difficult to determine whether this model indicates emotional problems and fear of commitment or actual personal growth.

Cohabiting

Living together as unmarried lovers has gone from being scandalous to normative in the United States in less than a generation. Couples cohabit for many reasons, including convenience, a trial marriage, and a permanently committed arrangement in which, for emotional or economic reasons, a pair chooses to avoid a legal marriage contract. The median length of cohabitation in the United States is 1.3 years, and 59% of these arrangements end in marriage (Graefe and Lichter 1999). Cohabiting couples have both the advantages and the disadvantages of a looser relational contract, including a sense of freedom, aliveness, and uncertainty. Although the basic tasks of couple coalition (e.g., dealing with intimacy, power, boundaries, sexuality) are present as in married couples, by definition cohabitation implies more permeable boundaries with the outside world, as well as some agreement on beliefs about permanence—for example, what their status means. Approximately 40% of cohabiting couples live with children from one or both partners in a *stepfamily* (Issacs and Leon 1988). Some research (Issacs and Leon 1988) suggests that living with a biological parent and that parent's lover is an extremely difficult situation for children, who are asked to relate to a person who may leave them and has no real rights to discipline or parent them yet cannot be ignored. Some evidence suggests that both physical and sexual abuses are more likely with a biologically unrelated adult in the house. When possible, cohabiting with children from former relationships in the house should be limited to permanent or soon-to-be-married couples.

Marital Separation

Separation is a relatively common crisis of marital life. Although it is emotionally traumatic for the individuals involved, it can serve as an opportunity to reassess the marital contract and individual goals. Separation in the early stages of a marriage may be caused by the partners coming down from their infatuation high, with subsequent disillusionment and eagerness to flee from the task of working things out. For those who married because of pregnancy, later recriminations about the reasons for the marriage may bring about a stormy period. Some people get married to get away from their parents' home or out of despair that they will ever be able to attract anyone else who will be seriously interested in them. When these underlying motives lose their force, the foundation of the marriage may be undermined. There are many other reasons for separation, including severe psychological problems in one or both partners, incompatibility, and extramarital affairs.

For some couples, differences in adult development lead to a situation in which two people no longer have much in common. Spouses whose children are grown and have left home may not easily become accustomed to living alone together as a marital couple. With the parental role diminished or absent, there may be little emotional or functional viability left in the marriage.

Although it is natural to think of marital separation as an unfortunate event, separation and its subsequent resolution can be considered as offering the potential for growth and change for the better. It offers a couple the opportunity to examine their relationship objectively. At the same time, the individuals can test their ability to adapt to living alone. This separation, together with new life experiences of various sorts, often enables the husband and wife to change their behaviors and feelings toward each other by the time they attempt reconciliation. If the couple are unable to communicate with each other or to learn about themselves, the separation will not be of much help, regardless of whether the couple reconcile. Clinical experience suggests that about half of couples who separate get back together. About half of those couples divorce later on (H.E. Kaplan and L. Epstein, personal communication, 1980).

Divorce

The divorce rate in most industrialized countries has been rising, although since the mid-1980s, it has shown signs of leveling off. If a marital relationship is old enough for true attachment to have taken place (about 2 years is usually considered long enough), divorce is one of the most painful experiences in anyone's life. We include a discussion of divorce here because on many occasions divorce is a positive step in an individual's or a family's life development. Many divorces are initiated when one partner is abusive, whether physically, sexually, or verbally. Ending such a union is often part of a maturation process.

Divorce is a process rather than an event and is characterized by its own developmental path. In fact, it usually represents one in a series of transitions that began with marital dissatisfaction and may or may not end with remarriage. A number of authors (Bohannan 1973; Kessler 1975; Salts 1979) have delineated stages of divorce, which are shown in Table 2–5.

TABLE 2–5.   **Stages of the divorce process**

---

1. The predivorce phase, involving growing disillusionment and dissatisfaction with the marriage and arrival at some consideration of divorce.
2. The separation itself, including moving out of the house and dealing with immediate grief. For many people this a period of great emotional distress, confusion, and grief—"crazy time."
3. The divorce, which typically occurs over the next 1–2 years. During this period, each member of the former couple deals with reorganizing his or her life structure, parenting issues, financial and family reorganization, community status, and legal issues.
4. For each former spouse, reforming of identity from part of a couple to single person (the psychic divorce). Couples who have children must find ways to remain connected as parents while separating as partners.

Although for some couples a divorce is mutual and relatively free of guilt, in most couples one member wants the divorce far more than the other does. Usually the rejected party feels enormously wounded and hurt, and the rejector often reacts with guilt and is therefore unable to mourn the very real losses. Later reactions may include fierce fighting over custody of children, money, or the story of what went wrong—this fighting may serve the purpose of punishment or revenge or may be a way of staying connected to the spouse. For many spouses, attachment (needing to know where the other person is, feeling secure in the other's presence) may last long after love or respect is gone, leading to confusing attempts to reconnect. The process of coming to grips with oneself, recognizing one's own part in the marital dissolution, and beginning to date again are often very anxiety provoking.

The Functional Single-Parent Family

One of the most dramatic social statistics of the 1990s was the increase in single-parent families. These are defined as family units in which there is only one parent because of defath, divorce, separation, or births outside marriage. In a single-parent family that has resulted from divorce, the other biological parent is often available and involved. These are often referred to as *binuclear families*, and in them child rearing is still a shared responsibility, even in different households. In 90% of families in which one parent has sole or almost sole responsibility for the children, this parent is the woman; about 10% of all families are one-parent families (U.S. Census Bureau 1997). Single-parent families share similar characteristics but may present a variety of different issues depending on whether there is another adult in residence, such as a grandparent or a lover, or whether the parent and child(ren) are alone in the house and answerable only to each other.

Single-parent households formed after a divorce or a death undergo a period of transition in which family structures have to be completely rethought out and reformed. Depending on the needs of the remaining parent, there may be a period of chaos before the basic tasks of providing food, shelter, organization, and discipline are reorganized. Evaluation of the impact of an absent spouse on the rest of the family unit must take into account the phase of family development in which the absence occurred, the length of the absence, the feelings of the remaining family members about the nonpresent member, and the mechanisms the family has used in coping with its changed constellation.

At first, all of this may seem overwhelming. After a time, however, the family unit may have reorganized itself and reached a new equilibrium. Binuclear families may face the task of dealing with two parents who are angry with each other and must collaborate, each of whom may have different child-rearing styles. Single-parent families in which the father is the head of the household appear to do just as well as those in which the mother is the main figure. Being the only parent, or the only custodial or residential parent, creates family issues that may include those shown in Table 2–6.

There are still many questions about whether identity formation is more difficult and love relationships more complicated for children of divorce, or whether the somewhat increased incidence of problems in these individuals is due to acrimonious divorce and financial stress. Regardless of whether the children of divorce have increased problems, however, a two-parent home that is affectionate, nonconflictual, and stable is still the easiest arrangement for both parents and children.

TABLE 2–6. **Family issues for single-parent families**

Social isolation and loneliness of the parent

Possible awkwardness in dating and jealousy on the part of the children

Demand by small children for the continuous physical presence of the sole parent

Children fending for themselves and carrying a greater share of the domestic responsibilities because the sole parent is working

Children feeling different from other children because they are members of a single-parent family

Less opportunity for a parent to discuss pros and cons of decisions and to get support and feedback when decisions are made

Crises and shifts caused by the introduction of a potential new mate or companion

---

Father-Headed Single-Parent Families

Thirteen percent of fathers are awarded sole custody of their children at the time of divorce (Friedman 1980), most often in cases where the mothers are deemed incompetent or male adolescent children are involved, although in some cases the mothers have left to pursue their careers or another relationship. Other father-headed families result from the wife's death, a highly traumatic event for everyone. More divorced men are demanding the right to custody of their children. Noncustodial mothers are more apt than noncustodial fathers to maintain contact with their children. Many American children under age 18 (many of them preschool age) now live with their male parents, and the numbers are increasing. With many more men taking over instrumental roles in parenting, fathers are arguing that they are just as capable and as indispensable to a child's development as are mothers.

In general, most fathers are much less comfortable in assuming custody of children than are mothers. This is due to the fact that, even now, most child-rearing and domestic roles are parceled out to mothers. After the initial period of apprehension, however, fathers seem capable of assuming the nurturing role as effectively as can mothers (Friedman 1980). To the extent that both parents can achieve collaboration (although living apart), the adjustment of the children will tend to be positive.

Binuclear Families

If both parents are interested in being involved in child rearing after divorce, the question of sharing time and decision making is crucial. Since the 1970s, many questions have arisen over the issue of the child's residence. Originally, the legal axiom "in the best interest of the child" proposed that one parent should have full charge of all custody and decision-making. It was shown that this arrangement led consistently to higher degrees of complete noninvolvement by the noncustodial parent, usually the father. When parents agree, joint legal custody has become the generally accepted arrangement in many states. However, this means only equal decision-making power in the eyes of the law. Joint physical custody, in which the child spends an approximately equal amount of time in both parents' homes, has both advantages and disadvantages. The many ways of setting up joint (physical) custody include, when geographically feasible, having children alternate the weeks or the days in which they visit either parent. Despite the objection that such an arrangement will confuse and upset the children, it appears that for some children this is an acceptable solution.

The most important issue for the children may be to have ongoing regular contact with each of their parents; this advantage may outweigh the disadvantages of having two homes. However, if the parents cannot find a way to parent amicably, the sense of disloyalty to each parent and the chaos of moving between two very different lifestyles is very hard on children, and single residential custody with ample visitation should be reconsidered.

Remarriage and the Remarried Family (Stepfamilies)

Becoming a remarried family requires a complex set of developmental adjustments that take several years to gel (Visher and Visher 1996). Family tasks for remarried families include forming a new parental coalition, establishing new traditions, negotiating different developmental needs, and developing a system that allows for many continuing shifts in household composition and within the larger system.

We define a stepfamily as a household in which there are two adults, at least one of whom has a child by a previous relationship (Visher and Visher 1996). The number of stepfamilies in the population is closely linked to the divorce rate, which has more than tripled since 1972. About 65% of these couplings involve children from prior marriages, and thus stepfamilies are formed. Demographers predict that, by 2010, stepfamilies will be the most common type of family (Visher and Visher 1996).

There are important differences in structure between stepfamilies and other types of families. These differences are generally not well understood by those in stepfamily situations and often lead to high stress during the early phases of integrating stepfamilies into a functioning unit (Visher and Visher 1996). Each of these structural differences imposes certain tasks on stepfamily members, and these tasks must be mastered before successful integration can occur. Table 2–7 presents a list of many of the tasks faced by stepfamilies.

TABLE 2–7. **Tasks for stepfamilies**

There are many losses and changes with which families must deal effectively.

There are incongruent individual marital and family life cycles that must be negotiated. For example, if a 50-year-old man with two grandchildren marries a 35-year-old woman with two young children, he may be a grandfather, a new husband, and a new father all at once.

Children and adults all come with a history of experiences and convictions from previous families about what is right and wrong, which may lead to differences of opinion that must be resolved so that new traditions can be established.

Parent-child relationships predate the new-couple relationship, so that a solid couple bond and new relationships with others in the stepfamily must be consciously developed.

There is a biological parent elsewhere in actuality or in memory, which challenges new stepfamily members to work out cooperative parenting relationships.

Children are often members of two households, and everyone must learn to deal with shifting household composition and complicated relationships. Children are frequently caught in loyalty conflicts.

There is little or no legal relationship between the stepparent and stepchildren; there is therefore a perceived risk in forming new relationships with little legal and societal support.

The dynamics of stepfamily life are different from those in traditional families. These differences are often insufficiently understood, thus depriving stepfamily members of needed information, education, and support. Many stepfamily members who lack information about these issues decide prematurely to dissolve their new relationship before the rewards and satisfactions of stepfamily life can become apparent.

Grandparent-Headed Families

In situations in which both parents have died or a single parent has become incapacitated by drugs or illness, children are often taken care of by grandparents. This has become more common in certain inner-city areas in which AIDS and crack cocaine have taken a major toll. The incongruent developmental needs of an aging person with those of an active young child, in addition to grief over the parental absence, make this system difficult but viable. Therapy tasks include determining the role of the parent in the child's life and maintaining social and financial support for the grandparents.

Gay and Lesbian Families

More gay and lesbian families are demanding the right to have their children from former marriages with them, to adopt children, or in the case of lesbians, to bear children within the union. These families face several unique tasks, including defining the legal and emotional roles of the nonbiological parent and dealing with the effects of homophobia on the child and the family. There is no evidence that these families produce a higher proportion of homosexual or problematic children.

■ REFERENCES

Bohannan P: The six stations of divorce, in Love, Marriage and Family: A Developmental Approach. Edited by Laswell ME, Lasswell TE. Chicago, IL, Scott, Foresman and Co., 1973

Duvall E: Family Development. Philadelphia, Lippincott, 1967, pp 44–46

Feldstein M, Rait D: Family assessment in an oncology setting. Cancer Nursing 15:161–172, 1990

Friedman HJ: The father's parenting experience in divorce. Am J Psychiatry 137:177–182, 1980

Gottman JM, Levenson RW: What predicts change in marital interaction over time? a study of alternative models. Fam Process 38:142–158, 1999

Graefe D, Lichter D: Life course transitions of American children: parental profile. Family Relations 38:24–28, 1989

Issacs M, Leon G: Remarriage and its alternatives following divorce: mother and child adjustment. J Marital Fam Ther 14:163–173, 1988

Kessler S: The American Way of Divorce: Prescription for Change. Chicago, IL, Nelson-Hall, 1975

Landeen J, Whelton C, Dermer S, et al: Needs of well siblings of persons with schizophrenia. Hosp Community Psychiatry 43:266–269, 1992

Lewis JM: For better or worse: interpersonal relationship and individual outcome. Am J Psychiatry 155:582–589, 1998

Reiss D, Plomin R, Hetherington M: Genetics and psychiatry: an unheralded window on the environment. Am J Psychiatry 148:283–291, 1991

Salts CJ: Divorce process: integration of theory. J Divorce 2:233–240, 1979.

Talan J: Living happily ever after? Newsday, April 12, 1988

Thomas V, Olson D: Problem families and the Circumplex Mode: observational assessment using the Clinical Rating Scale (CRS). J Marital Fam Ther 19:159–176, 1993

U.S. Census Bureau: Statistical abstract of the United States. Washington, DC, U.S. Government Printing Office, 1997

Visher EB, Visher JS: Therapy with stepfamilies. New York, Brunner/Mazel, 1996

Walsh F: Conceptualizations of normal family processes, in Normal Family Processes, 2nd Edition. Edited by Walsh F. New York, Guilford, 1993, p 45

3

DYSFUNCTIONAL FAMILIES

■ CURRENT PERSPECTIVES

In the preceding chapters, we describe the organization and behavior of the functional family, using the concept of the family as a system with its own life cycles and tasks. In this chapter, we focus on the disturbances in these areas and the ways in which families become dysfunctional. We discuss the types of disturbances manifested by dysfunctional family systems, including problematic family beliefs and myths, individual symptomatology, life cycle stressors, and the inability of the family to accomplish family tasks.

How do problems develop? What leads to symptoms? Who begins to realize that a problem is distressing enough to require outside intervention? These are issues that intrigue family theorists and preoccupy the family therapist as he or she begins the assessment of a couple or family.

Family systems explanations for symptoms are as numerous as schools of clinical theory and practice, yet there are a small group of hypotheses that seem to be commonly endorsed (Table 3–1). The strongest predictor of overall life satisfaction is the quality of a person's central relationship. In addition, "a good and stable relationship buffers against the genetic vulnerability to both medical and psychiatric disorders" (J.M. Lewis, personal communication, May 1998; see Lewis 1998 for full discussion of this issue).

TABLE 3–1. **Family system explanations for symptoms**

Symptoms:

May emerge as a result of problematic communication or interactional patterns in a family

May signal impasse at a particular developmental point in the family's life cycle

May be part of solution behavior that is failing at its task

May reflect problems in family structure and organization

May be expressed when aspects of a family's life are denied or dissociated

May represent a lack of validation

May be an expression of an underlying medical or psychiatric illness

May simply relate to misfortune and bad luck

■ STRUCTURAL PROBLEMS

Sometimes the symptoms in an individual may be viewed as a reflection of organizational problems existing within the marriage or the family. According to Minuchin (1974), family structure is

> the invisible set of functional demands that organizes the ways in which family members interact. A family is a system that operates through transactional patterns. Repeated transactions establish patterns of how, when, and to whom to relate, and these patterns underpin the system. (p. 51)

In Minuchin's influential structural approach, a pathological family could be one that "in the face of stress increases the rigidity of their transactional patterns and boundaries, and avoids or resists any exploration of alternatives" (p. 55). As the family's range of choices narrows, family members develop predictable and stereotyped responses to each other and to the extrafamilial environment. In turn, the family becomes a closed system, and family members experience themselves as controlled and impotent (Papp 1980). From the structural perspective, then, the family therapist's definition of a pathogenic family is one whose adaptive and coping mechanisms have been exhausted. Symptoms or unhappiness in a family member are embedded in the problematic family function.

Dimensions of family structure that warrant attention are family boundaries, hierarchy, and coalitions. As discussed in Chapter 1, Minuchin (1974) considers boundaries on a continuum ranging from enmeshment to disengagement. *Enmeshment* refers to a style of family involvement in which boundaries within the family are highly permeable, but those between the family and outside are usually rigid. In more disengaged families, only a high level of stress can reverberate strongly enough to activate the family's supportive systems (e.g., serious illness or a suicide attempt). If boundaries address proximity, the dimension of hierarchy is defined in terms of authority or relative influence that family members exercise in relation to one another.

Problems in alliances or coalitions represent another facet of structural difficulties. In a three-person system, there are ample opportunities for two to be allied against the third member. Minuchin (1974) has described three different types of triangles:

1. Triangulation, in which parents make equally strong but different demands on the child, who responds with paralysis (unable to choose), by moving back and forth between parents (go-between), or with rebellion
2. Detouring, in which parental conflict is put aside to attend to the child, either to care for her because she is needy or ill (protective) or to attack her because she is misbehaving (hostile and blaming); this requires that the child continue to be problematic so that parents can avoid the conflict
3. Stable coalition between one parent and a child, in which a parent and child are closely tied, either in response to the other parent's underinvolvement or to block the other parent's involvement

Problems in family structure can be likened to structural problems in a house: if problems are left unattended to, symptoms gradually emerge and can worsen.

■ THE SOLUTION AS THE PROBLEM

In the model described here, symptoms are explained not by faults in each person but by problems in the rules of the systems or patterns of repetitive interaction. All families are faced with everyday problems in living—how to get household tasks completed, how to get children to go to school and do their homework, how to compromise when differences occur. In facing a problem, each family member tends to approach a problem in characteristic ways of thinking, feeling, and acting. These initial responses may or may not be effective for the specific problem. If the family members are unable to modify the problem-solving behavior when it does not work, they may continue to repeat the same ineffective behavior to the point that a small problem turns into a major one.

> Mrs. A believed that children should eat specific kinds and amounts of food. When her son did not do this, she punished him. The oldest child, a compliant boy with a good appetite, responded by eating in the way she required. The younger child, however, was temperamentally more of a fighter and had an uncertain appetite. He refused to eat. Mrs. A continued to apply the same problem-solving behavior of punishment, and the result was a pitched battle and eventually an eating disorder.

This model posits that mishandling of the original problem occurs when 1) a solution is attempted by denying that a problem is a problem and doing nothing, 2) change is attempted for something that is unchangeable or nonexistent, or 3) action is taken at the wrong level (Watzlawick et al. 1974).

Sometimes the problem is a conflict in problem-solving behaviors between family members. For example, a child stays home for a week with the flu. Her mother, who is lonely and bored, is happy to have her at home. When the child has recovered from the flu, she protests and says she is still sick. Her mother wants to keep her home, and her father says that her mother is spoiling her and that she must go to school. The argument raises the child's anxiety, and she throws up and is allowed to stay home. Eventually she develops a school phobia. If this process results in the child forming a coalition with the mother against the father, the problem has changed the family structure.

Sometimes the problem is real but the solution is ineffective. For example, when a husband began drinking, his wife tried to protect him by covering for him, calling in sick for him, and so forth. This behavior allowed him to continue his drinking, and she became depressed by the situation. When she no longer supported him and said that she would leave him if the behavior continued, she became less depressed and he also stopped drinking. When the attempted solution becomes the problem, the way to change the situation is to do something else.

■ FAMILY BELIEFS AND MYTHS

Individuals and families have belief systems that, in part, determine their feelings and behaviors. These subterranean structures have been referred to as *family myths*. They are often found to be important contributors and maintainers of family difficulty, and family therapists must be aware of them if they are to understand family behavior. For example, in the case above, the wife's belief that a good woman must stand by her man made it impossible for her to stop covering for her husband. Only when she became depressed and he lost his job from alcoholism was she able to change her belief to "In the end you cannot allow another person to destroy your life" and to set some limits. Ferreira (1963) defines family myths as "a series of fairly well integrated beliefs shared by all family members, concerning each other and their mutual position in the family, which go unchallenged by everyone involved, in spite of the reality distortions which they may conspicuously imply" (p. 457). The implications of Ferreira's definition involve very personalized and specific myths for each family, in which individual family members are singled out for particular roles or self-fulfilling prophecies, such as "Mother is the emotional one in the family" or "our son misbehaves continually."

In addition to specific family myths, a variety of myths are promulgated by the culture. Many of these are therefore shared by family members and perhaps by the therapist. The therapist must be sensitive to and deal with those beliefs that seem to be deleterious to a family's functioning and, conversely, must understand that some myths aid functioning. Some examples of myths or beliefs are shown in Table 3–2.

The common denominator of these myths is the idea that there is some substitute for the slow, painful, but ultimately exciting work of knowing the partner as a separate person and oneself as a person with separate ideas and needs for aloneness and togetherness. Everyone needs positive feedback, and no one can read minds well enough to substitute for clear communication. Separation and divorce may or may not be best for the children and may or may not be a failure of the individual (although it feels like one to most people).

■ THE LARGER SOCIAL SYSTEM AND DYSFUNCTION

Systems theory encompasses not only the family but also the wider community. The family is basically a subsystem of the community and culture in which it is embedded.

Often the surrounding culture puts enormous pressure on the family system. The fit between the family and the culture, in certain locations or in cases of immigration, may be problematic. For example, the only Jewish family living in an anti-Semitic small town may develop boundaries that in another situation would be called enmeshed, but in this case are necessary to protect the children. A couple in an arranged marriage with a very traditional role structure who comes to the United States can be torn apart if the woman is the only partner able to get a job and be out in the new culture.

Traditional gender roles also overdetermine family life. A family with an overinvolved mother and distant father is not just a family with problems, it is the end result of a historical and cultural pattern in which men are encouraged to see their worth as economic and women are seen as the children's caregivers.

TABLE 3–2. **Family myths**

If life has not worked out well for you as an individual, getting married will make everything better.

Marital and family life should be totally happy, and each individual therein should expect either all or most gratifications to come from the family system.

Marital partners should be completely honest with one another at all times.

A happy marriage is one in which there are no disagreements, and when family members fight with one another, it means that they hate each other.

Marital partners should be as unselfish as possible and give up thinking about their own individual needs.

When something goes wrong in the family, one should look around to see who is at fault.

When things are not going well, it will often be of help to spend a major part of the time digging up past as well as present hurts.

In a marital argument one partner is right and the other is wrong, and the goal of such fights should be for the partners to see who can score the most points.

A good sexual relationship will inevitably lead to a good marriage.

Marital partners increasingly understand each other's verbal and nonverbal communications, so there is little or no need to check things with one another.

Positive feedback is not as necessary in marital systems as is negative feedback.

"And then they lived happily ever after."

Any spouse can (and should) be reformed and remodeled into the shape desired by the partner.

Everyone knows what a husband should be like and what a wife should be like.

If a marriage is not working properly, having children will rescue it.

No matter how bad the marriage, it should be kept together for the sake of the children.

If the marriage does not work, an extramarital affair or a new marriage will cure the situation.

Separation and divorce represent a failure of the marriage and of the individuals involved.

■ COMMENTARY: THE DEVELOPMENT OF SYMPTOMS IN A PARTICULAR PERSON

Marital and family systems, like individuals, have characteristic patterns of coping with stress. The family's first line of defense is usually to evoke and strengthen adaptive patterns that the family has used in the past. If these are maladaptive, the type of disturbance that results may be similar to the inflexible character of an individual with a personality disorder.

If characteristic adaptive mechanisms are not available or fail to deal adequately with the situation, one or another family member may develop overt symptoms. These symptoms in the family member may cause the individual to be labeled bad or sick. The appropriate social helping institutions may become involved with that individual in an attempt to deal with the particular symptomatic expression. The individual then takes on the role of the *identified patient*. More often than not, the family context from which the individual's symptoms emanate is overlooked or inadequately attended to. The so-called bad, sick, or crazy family member is treated and is found either intractable or improved. If improved, he or she may soon become symptomatic again when returned to the family context or may cause another family member to become symptomatic. The underlying family disturbance will have to be treated. Often the symptom bearer is biologically vulnerable.

A major tenet of family therapists, therefore, is that the symptomatic family member is often thought of as being indicative of widespread disturbance in the entire family system (Ackerman 1958; Bateson et al. 1956; Bell 1961; Carroll 1960; Counts 1967). If the therapist overlooks or deals inadequately with the more general family disturbance, family members are likely to continue to be symptomatic.

The patterns of interaction within a family cannot always be clearly related to any specific dysfunction. The reasons why a specific type of disturbance is manifested in a family system or member are not understood clearly at present, but certain innate tendencies and life circumstances probably favor the development of one or another symptomatic expression in a particular instance.

Similarly, the reasons why one family member rather than another becomes symptomatic have not been definitively settled. A number of reasons, however, have been given to account for this phenomenon. These reasons are shown in Table 3–3.

TABLE 3–3. **Reasons a family member may become symptomatic**

Individual susceptibility, that is, genetic predisposition: For example, an individual who was born brain damaged and is under family stress is likely to become symptomatic. Inborn temperamental differences may contribute (Thomas and Chess 1985). Likewise, biological disposition to an Axis I disorder like schizophrenia, bipolar disorder, attention-deficit/hyperactivity disorder, or a learning disorder in a child also creates increased vulnerability to illness.

Situation in the family at the time of birth: For example, a parent whose own parent died around the time of the birth of a child might use the newborn infant to work out his feelings about his own dead parent.

Physical illness of the child: A child who is chronically ill may have family problems projected on him whenever he has an acute episode. In addition, the amount of care needed by the ill child may skew family function, leading to infantilization of the ill child as well as anger and resentment in well siblings.

Precipitant in the extended family: Accidents or a death that relates somehow to one child more than another (e.g., an eldest daughter who was with her grandmother the day the grandmother had a heart attack) may make one family member the focus for family problems.

The sex of a child may correspond to a particular difficulty of the parent. For example, if a father feels particularly inadequate with other males, his son may become symptomatic.

Birth order of siblings: The eldest child may get the major parental loading, whereas the youngest child is often babied and kept dependent.

Family myth attached to a specific individual: Certain people in families are known, for example, as the stupid one, the smart one, the lazy one, the good-looking one, and the ugly one. First names of children and nicknames may reveal these myths. A child is sometimes named after a godparent or other person who is significant in the parents' past and, in turn, carries a myth attached to that person.

It has been suggested that in less than optimal families, the mother is the first to suffer from the system's inadequacy. She is most often the first to become distressed or symptomatic. At increased levels of family system dysfunction, a child may also begin to experience distress and become symptomatic. In many cases, he or she will then become an identified patient. The father, who traditionally has more in the way of outside sources of esteem, is often the last family member to become symptomatic (Lewis et al. 1976).

The symptomatic family member may be the family scapegoat, on whom family difficulties are displaced, or may be psychologically or constitutionally the weakest, the youngest, or the most sensitive family member. The identified patient may be the family member who is most interested or involved in the process of changing the family. For example, some teenagers want to "save" their parents because they are not getting along with each other. One hypothesis about family functioning is that these children may begin to steal in order to get caught so that the entire family can be referred for help.

■ LIFE CYCLE PROBLEMS AND DYSFUNCTION

Although some families continually struggle with problems over their lives, others experience difficulties only during specific life cycle periods. A family is subject to inner pressure from developmental changes in its own members and subsystems and to outer pressure from demands to accommodate to the significant social institutions that have an impact on its members. Episodic family problems may be related to 1) an inability to cope adequately with the tasks of the current family phase, 2) the need to move on to a new family phase, and/or 3) the stress of unexpected, idiosyncratic events.

In the case of normal, expectable family life crises, a family's inability to master the present tasks may be the cause for the expression of symptoms. For example, two people optimally need to reach a certain stage in their own personal development, as well as in their relationships with their family of origin, before being ready, as two independent individuals, to consider marriage. To the extent that this and other prior stages are not successfully mastered, the individuals and the marital unit will be hampered in dealing with current challenges. This same hypothesis can be applied to each of the family phases, wherein a family's skill at a particular stage may not necessarily transfer to similar capacities at the next developmental stage. Although expected developmental transitions may be stressful for family members, unexpected or idiosyncratic changes can also be difficult to handle. Unusual events in the family life cycle may overwhelm the coping capacities of family systems. Common examples of such events are unemployment, catastrophic illness, accidents, violent crime, or a death in the family. Marital and family systems, like individuals, have characteristic patterns of coping with stress. The family's first line of defense is usually to evoke and strengthen characteristic adaptive patterns that the family has used in the past. If these responses rigidly constrain experimentation and a flexible reaction, the type of disturbance may be similar to its analogue in individual terms—the inflexible character of an individual with a rigid personality style.

Whatever the particulars of a family's dysfunction, outlining the family's individual life cycle aids in elucidating their idiosyncrasies, as well as providing a framework from which successful therapy can begin (Carter and McGoldrick 1988).

Unresolved Grief

A death in the family of a parent or a child commonly leads to family problems, especially when mourning does not occur. Often the family's development stops at the point of the death and the family remains in limbo, unable to move on or to truly grieve. This is often expressed in family ritual—for example, if a child dies near Christmas, the family may be unable to celebrate for years to come or may insist that the Christmas ritual be exactly the same as before the child died, long past the point where the ritual would have changed to accommodate the other children. Death from stillbirth or miscarriage may have the same effect. Most often the family needs to talk about the death, to find some way to grieve, and to be given permission to continue living.

Toxic Secrets

Families may have secrets that some members know but others do not (for example, the mother and the daughter, but not the father, may know that the daughter was raped), that everyone knows but no one admits (Dad is alcoholic), or that most people are aware of or strongly suspect but do not acknowledge (Mom is having an affair). Secrets prevent clear communication, skew coalitions, and mystify children who know something is wrong but not what. Secrets contribute an air of unreality to the family, which is generally considered to impede a child's development and reality testing.

The therapist must find a way to open the secret carefully, giving time to support everyone in the family. It is seldom in the family's best interest for people to keep a major family secret.

■ TASK PERFORMANCE IN THE DYSFUNCTIONAL FAMILY

Various deficiencies in carrying out the family's functions will lead to strains, distortions, problems, and symptoms in family life. The major family tasks are to provide for the members' basic physical requirements, to develop a working marital coalition, and to rear the offspring. In the dysfunctional family, these tasks are either not handled or handled differently and less adaptively than in healthy families. Task performance in the family may be compromised by an unendurable environment, by a physical or mental illness of one or more family members, or by serious conflict among family members, particularly the marital dyad or adult caregivers.

Supporting Physical Needs of Members

Inability to support the family's physical needs in particular must be considered in situations of war, poverty, or economic depression. Maintaining family integrity in the face of severe poverty requires ingenuity and endurance. However, inability to provide for basic material needs may occur in the face of adequate finances if the caregiving adults are "absent" because of drug or alcohol addiction, psychosis, violence, or being so caught up in their own concerns that they are oblivious to those in their care.

Issues of Sex, Intimacy, and Commitment: Maintaining a Functional Marriage

Marriage is one of the few human relationships that functions on two levels—as a love relationship and as a functional economic partnership. It therefore requires a complex set of skills and the ability to switch from one functioning mode to another. It is possible to have a marriage in which intimacy is absent but in which the couple functions well, as "roommates," to parent and keep the home going. It is also possible to have a marriage in which sex and passion are very much present but in which fierce battles over power and control issues make it difficult or impossible to get much done. As the couple become more dysfunctional, anger and rage overwhelm positive feelings, communication, and task completion, leaving the couple either in a constant battle or with one spouse completely dominating the other.

Rearing and Socialization of Children

It is difficult to deal with the constant needs of children when one is overwhelmed by marital strife, individual illness or addiction, or racism and poverty. The more parents are disconnected from the part of themselves that is capable of nurturing, the more the child is neglected or used to take care of the parents by being held responsible for either household tasks or emotional support of a parent. The ultimate form of this is incest, in which the child becomes a substitute sexual object. Children as young as age 4 or 5 can be inducted into trying to cheer up a depressed parent, making their own meals because the parents have forgotten, or trying to shield a younger child from abuse.

Members of dysfunctional families may demonstrate styles of thinking and communication that are particularly difficult for children, including intrusive, projective, or bizarre thinking. In some families the children's emotions are consistently denied, contradicted, ignored, or punished, leading to depression, rage, or numbing in the children.

It needs to be said, however, that some children are very difficult to deal with, and the task of child rearing can be formidable. Children with a difficult temperament or some form of brain damage such as attention-deficit/hyperactivity disorder, autism, or pervasive developmental disorder or some forms of child psychosis require extraordinary reserves of patience and attention. The parent of such a child must maintain a calm, structured environment in the face of constant testing. If the parents do not share a commitment to put in extra time or if they cannot reach agreement on ways of dealing with the child, these children can cause major rifts in marriages that otherwise would function within the normal range. Other children might not be difficult for both parents but temperamentally are a bad fit with one parent. For example, a very active, mischievous boy might be a bad match for a fearful and depressed mother, who might deal better with a more docile and quiet child; or a boy who is shy and retiring might be a great disappointment to a demanding, athletic father who may try to toughen him up by being harsh in a way that leaves permanent scars.

■ REFERENCES

Ackerman N: Psychodynamics of family life, diagnosis and treatment in family relationships. New York, Basic Books, 1958

Bateson G, Jackson D, Haley J, Weakland J: Toward a theory of schizophrenia. Behav Sci 1:251–254, 1956

Bell JE: Family group therapy. Public Health Monograph No. 64. Washington, DC: U.S. Department of Health, Education and Welfare, Public Health Service, 1961

Carroll EJ: Treatment of the family as a unit. Pa Med 63:57–62, 1960

Carter B, McGoldrick M: Conceptual overview, in The Changing Family Life Cycle: A Framework for Family Therapy, 2nd Edition. Edited by Carter B, McGoldrick M. New York, Gardner Press, 1988, pp 3–25

Counts R: Family crisis and the impulsive adolescent. Arch Gen Psychiatry 17:74, 1967

Ferreira AJ: Family myths and homeostasis. Arch Gen Psychiatry 9:457–463, 1963

Lewis JM: For better or worse: interpersonal relationships and individual outcome. Am J Psychiatry 155:582–589, 1998

Lewis JM, Beavers WR, Gossett JT, et al: No Single Thread: Psychological Health in Family Systems. New York, Brunner/Mazel, 1976

Minuchin S: Families and Family Therapy. Cambridge, MA, Harvard University Press, 1974

Papp P: The Process of Change. New York, Guilford, 1980

Thomas A, Chess S: Temperament and Development. New York, Guilford, 1985

Watzlawick P, Weakland J, Fisch R: Change: Principles of Problem Formation and Problem Resolution. New York, WW Norton, 1974

4

CONDUCTING A
FAMILY EVALUATION

The evaluation of a married couple or a family should be understood as a continuing process that is begun at the first contact but not necessarily completed at any particular point. Some initial formulation, such as an understanding of what is wrong, is useful to the therapist to help with the marshaling of data and forming of hypotheses, but in a larger sense, the evaluation is often an inextricable part of the therapy itself. If patients can hear and analyze their histories, their present situations will change.

As data are gathered, the therapist forms hypotheses based on a conceptual frame of reference. The therapist should assign priorities and weight to the variety of contributory variables while setting up an overall intervention strategy. It is hoped that the particular intervention will lead to desired therapy goals. In this process, further data are obtained that serve to confirm, modify, or negate the original hypotheses, strategies, and tactics. These later formulations are then tested in the matrix of the family sessions as further data are obtained.

■ ROLE OF HISTORICAL MATERIAL

There are several points of view regarding the type and quantity of the historical data to be gathered during a family evaluation. Some family therapists begin with a specific and detailed longitudinal history of the family unit and its constituent members, which may perhaps span three or more generations—that is, the *genogram*. This method has the advantage of permitting the family and the therapist to review the complex background of the present situation together. The therapist will begin to understand unresolved past and present issues, will usually gain a sense of rapport and identification with the family and its members, and may then feel more comfortable in defining problem areas and in forming a strategy. The family benefits by reviewing together the source and evolution of its current condition, which may prove to be a clarifying, empathy-building process for the entire family. The good and the bad are brought into focus, and the immediate distress is placed in a broader perspective. Sometimes a family in crisis is too impatient to tolerate exhaustive history gathering, and therefore, in acute situations, lengthy data gathering must be curtailed.

Other therapists do not rely heavily on the longitudinal approach. They prefer to begin with a cross-sectional view of family functioning, delineating the situation that led the family to seek treatment at the present time. This cross-sectional view attempts to understand the current problem. This procedure has the advantage of starting with the problems about which the family is most concerned and is not as potentially time consuming or as seemingly remote from the present realities as the longitudinal method. The therapist, however, may not emerge with as sharp a focus on important family patterns because much of the discussion may be negatively tinged, owing to the family's preoccupation with its current difficulty.

A family's biography is an altered history bent through the prism of the telling person. History reported by the involved individuals must be considered as potentially biased, second-hand information, because the therapist is not directly witnessing the dysfunction being described. The information will vary widely with the historians, and key pieces of information may be omitted. This includes events that the reporter has no reason to believe are related to those childhood behaviors. In addition, because beliefs about an event or situation affect behavior, the person's story, accurate or not, is a crucial part of the person's history.

To a considerable extent, these differences in technique may mirror differences in the therapists' training, theoretical beliefs, and temperaments. Most therapists, however, probably use combinations of these approaches as the situation warrants, for there is no evidence of one technique being superior to the others. We recommend reviewing both past and present and constructing a two- or preferably three-generation genogram.

■ WHOM TO INCLUDE IN THE FAMILY EVALUATION

An early and strategic question is what members of the family to include in the evaluation sessions. In many cases, from the very first contact, often by phone call, the therapist talks to one individual, who represents the family and presents the problem. The problem may be presented as a family problem or as an individual's problem that is disturbing other family members. We assume here that, from the very first phone call or contact by a family member, the therapist is considering the possibility of family intervention or other types of intervention such as individual intervention, either alone or in combination with family therapy.

Thus, the question arises of whom to include in the evaluation sessions. Most family therapists would agree that it is important, from the first session, to include all members of the family in the evaluation sessions. This usually means all members of a nuclear family, that is, the mother, father, and children who reside under the same roof. Relatives living with the family should probably also be included at some point. In addition to nuclear family members (especially in new family forms), significant others must be included if they are living with or deeply involved with the children.

Clinical experience suggests that it is easier to include all family members for evaluation sessions at the beginning rather than waiting until later to do so. This allows a clearer picture of family dynamics and crystallization of family problems. If one begins with all family members, including the marital subsystem and the children subsystem, then one can have subsequent sessions with one subsystem while excluding the other.

There may be particular circumstances when one would not want to include the whole family in the evaluation sessions. For example, a couple who present with sexual difficulties should be seen as a couple without their children. Likewise, the couple may be seen alone for what they identify as marital difficulties without involving the children, although the children may be included later if appropriate. Many therapists will see both spouses together in an initial evaluation session, followed by an individual session with each spouse alone. Although some would say that such a situation encourages one spouse to tell secrets to the therapist, others suggest that the only way for a therapist to proceed is to have all information at the beginning. Some therapists use individual sessions with each spouse but indicate before the session that this is not confidential to the couple sessions, thus precluding the forming of coalitions and yet possibly discouraging the full disclosure of information.

A practical consideration that often arises is the issue of evaluation sessions when one or more central family members are absent. We believe that in many cases such missing family members are crucial to the problem, that their absence must be discussed, and that they should be brought in to the sessions. Napier and Whitaker (1978) give an interesting clinical illustration of a family in which the initial evaluation session is stopped because of a missing son and the family's task becomes to insist on his participation. It is probably not an uncommon practice of family therapists to refuse to proceed with the evaluation until the missing member is present. However, some therapists will conduct a few sessions without a missing member, focusing on how they could be convinced to come in as one of the issues of treatment. If, for example, a major family problem has been a couple's inability to put limits on their 16-year-old son, refusing to treat them until they bring him in would result in their giving up on treatment. A better move might be to make the focus of treatment with the couple a discussion of how they could set enough limits to produce him.

■ PROGRESSION OF THE FAMILY EVALUATION INTERVIEW

Several authors have discussed the sequential progression of the family evaluation interview (Haley 1976; Minuchin 1974). Most would suggest that the first interview task is to greet each of the family members and to begin to accommodate the family. This accommodation is accomplished by noting the power system of the family, acquiescing to it, and using the family vocabulary that surfaces. Next, the interview can proceed to some delineation of the family problem as each family member sees it.

Reiss (1981) has provided a helpful analysis of the choice points that a clinician faces in the initial assessment of a family. He distinguishes substantive or theoretical choice points from technical choice points.

The first substantive choice point is whether to focus on the cross-sectional, current functioning of the family or to give more attention to the longitudinal, developmental history of the family unit and its individuals, as discussed earlier in this chapter (see "Role of Historical Material" earlier in this chapter). A second choice point is whether to focus on the family as the central shaping force or on the environment or community (e.g., its forces and properties) that influence the family. The latter would include focus on the network of relatives and friends, the school, and so forth. A third choice point concerns crisis versus character orientation. The former is a focus on the current, immediate, concrete problem or symptom that brings the family in, whereas the latter is a focus on the more enduring patterns of self-protection, cognitive and affective style, and deficits that the family manifests. A fourth choice point is whether to focus on the pathology or the functional competence of the family unit. Each family will function well in some areas, not as well in others. A fifth choice point concerns the basic theoretical understanding of the evaluator and his or her emphasis on finding family themes versus looking at concrete behaviors and their consequences. In the psychoanalytic tradition, there is an emphasis on discovering the thematic or underlying (conscious or unconscious) structures that give family life and behavior its meaning and thrust. In contrast, therapists with a behavioral orientation focus on the problem behaviors and their antecedent and consequent events.

The first technical choice point concerns the pacing of the assessment. Some advocate a thorough assessment before beginning treatment, with a clear marker between, whereas others emphasize that assessment and treatment merge, especially as assessment involves making interventions and assessing how the family responds. A second choice point involves individualized measurement of the family (emphasizing the uniqueness of the family) or standardized measurement of the family, focusing on major dimensions that are relevant to all families. A third choice point involves assessing, the issue of dimensionalizing the data (how the family rates on communication, for example) or typologizing the family (the enmeshed family, for example). A fourth technical choice point is the clinician's perspective of being inside or emphatically feeling what it is like to be with this family versus observing, as objectively as possible (as an outsider), how the family performs and carries out functions. The fifth and sixth choice points are whether to focus on children or adults and whether the method should be talking or an activity.

These decision points are not either-or situations, of course, and the evaluation will emphasize different areas on the polar dimensions, depending on the situation. However, they are indeed choice points that must be faced in a time-limited setting of conducting evaluations.

For those fortunate enough to work in training centers or non-solo practices, one effective way of evaluating families is with a team behind a one-way mirror. The experience of being behind a mirror and watching is fundamentally different from being in the room—subtle emotional cues or anxiety or connection are often missed, but the overall pattern, including the relationship of therapist to family, are more clear. With a team, one can obtain many different viewpoints. It is humbling but valuable to see how the understanding of a family is affected by the personality, age, and gender of the viewer, and the process opens up many different realities for the therapist.

■ ROLE OF INDIVIDUAL AND FAMILY DIAGNOSIS

The decision of whom to include in the family evaluation raises the question of for what purpose individuals are to be included. The discussion here is based on our bias that both the family as a whole and the individuals in the family are important in the diagnostic equation.

In psychiatry, there is an imperfect relationship between individual diagnosis and treatment planning, because the diagnosis itself often does not give enough information to plan the interventions. This imperfect relationship is compounded in family therapy, where one must have enough information to make an individual diagnosis (especially if there is a clearly identified patient) and also to make a family diagnostic statement.

In assessing families, one must obtain enough individual information to be able to give individual DSM-IV-TR (American Psychiatric Association 2000) diagnoses to members with pathology that meets criteria. There is no central place in DSM-IV-TR for family pathology. However, there is a section called "Other Conditions That May Be a Focus of Clinical Attention" on Axis I. Subsumed (or embedded) in this section are "Relational Problems."

DSM-IV-TR clearly has a narrow limit of usefulness for many family therapists. From the point of view of the framers of that classification, the lack of any emphasis on the classification of family pathology in DSM-IV-TR may have been necessary, given both the purpose and individual orientation of DSM-IV-TR and the current lack of research evidence supporting various methods of classifying family pathology. We disagree and would argue that Axis IV, the rating of psychosocial stressors and environmental problems, may be most helpful in indicating patients for whom family problems are prominent. At present, although there are many proposed typologies of family functioning, we think that family typologizing is premature. Rather, the family diagnosis should consist of dimensional statements concerning the family and its functioning, as outlined in the family diagnostic outline in the next two chapters in this volume.

Of note, in preparation for DSM-V, a diagnostic classification for children is being developed. In that proposal, Axis II describes "symptomatic disorders specific to caregiver-child *relationships* [italics ours] based on the clinician's structured observation of the pairs interactions" (Emde 2001). Not all family therapists use DSM criteria, and we believe that individual family members must be assessed at least to determine the presence of serious psychopathology and the need for medication.

■ DIMENSIONS OF FAMILY FUNCTION

Because of its thoroughness, operational definitions, congruence with the major areas of family functioning or dysfunctioning mentioned previously, teachability, and relevance to treatment planning, we recommend a modified version of the McMaster model of family evaluation (Epstein and Bishop 1981). This model contains six dimensions of family functioning that must be assessed, dimensions that are congruent with the concepts of functional and dysfunctional families (enumerated in previous chapters) and with the consensus areas of importance across family models mentioned in the previous paragraph. These dimensions are communication, problem solving, roles and coalition, affective responsiveness, involvement, behavior control, and operative family beliefs and stories. In addition, the therapist must carefully evaluate the family members' beliefs about themselves and about the problem. Finally, the family's cultural background and its patterns of beliefs and values must be assessed.

■ OUTLINE FOR FAMILY EVALUATION

Drawing heavily from the McMaster evaluation model and integrating other aspects, we have developed the evaluation outline presented in Table 4–1. This outline offers a practical alternative to either gathering an extensive history or plunging into the middle of the family interaction. Although far from exhaustive in scope, this outline provides some anchoring points for initial understanding and planning. It is not meant to be inflexible or unchangeable, and it certainly can be expanded or contracted as the situation warrants.

TABLE 4–1.	**Family evaluation outline**

I. Gathering identifying data and establishing current phase of family life cycle

II. Gathering explicit interview data
   A. What is the current family problem?
   B. Why does the family come for treatment at the present time?
      1. Recent family events and stresses
   C. What is the background of the family problem?
   D. What is the history of past treatment attempts or other attempts at problem solving in the family? What other problems has the family had?
   E. What are the family's goals and expectations of the treatment? What are its strengths, motivations, and resistances?

III. Formulating the family problem areas
   A. Rating important dimensions of family functioning
      1. Communication
      2. Problem solving
      3. Roles and coalitions
      4. Affective responsiveness and involvement
      5. Behavior control
      6. Operative family beliefs and stories
   B. Family classification and diagnosis

IV. Planning the therapeutic approach and establishing the treatment contract

Source. Reprinted from Glick ID, Berman EM, Clarkin JF, et al: *Marital and Family Therapy,* 4th Edition, 2000, p. 153. Copyright 2000, American Psychiatric Press, Inc. Used with permission. Table includes material adapted from the McMaster model in Epstein and Bishop 1981; Gill et al. 1954; and Group for the Advancement of Psychiatry 1970.

■ CURRENT PHASE OF FAMILY LIFE CYCLE

Identifying Data

Family members' names, ages, relationships, family composition, ethnicity, socioeconomic status, and living arrangements should be obtained early. To identify the current phase of the family life cycle, the therapist should ascertain the ages and relationships of those family members living under one roof, adult children living separately, and ages of grandparents. An important criterion for understanding the family's structure is knowing each stage the family has reached in its developmental cycle. Each stage of the family life cycle has unique stresses, challenges, opportunities, and pitfalls. By being alert to these aspects, the therapist is in a position to observe and explore those particular tasks, roles, and relationships that are phase specific for the family. The therapist can also discover to what extent the family members clearly recognize and are attempting to cope with issues relevant to the family's current stage of development.

For many married couples and families, the basic difficulty underlying the need for professional help can be related to their inability to cope satisfactorily with their current developmental phase or to transition into the next one. The B family, mentioned later in this chapter, is a good example of the type of problem that arises in a later stage of marriage—the empty-nest syndrome—in which the parents could not cope with the separation of their children from the home, in part because of their fear of being alone as husband and wife.

One or both parents may be going through an individual developmental phase that powerfully affects the family life cycle. For example, a new baby born to a 40-year-old mother and a 60-year-old father may be in conflict with the father's sense of aging and his thoughts of ease and retirement. On the other hand, it might bring both parents a sense of renewed youth and empowerment.

■ EXPLICIT INTERVIEW DATA

What Is the Current Family Problem?

The interviewer asks each family member, in turn, with all family members present, what that individual believes to be the current problem in the family. The interviewer attempts to maintain the focus on the current family problem, rather than on one or another individual or on past difficulties. Each family member receives an equal opportunity to be heard, without interruption, and to feel that his or her opinions and views are worthwhile, important, and acknowledged. The interviewer will begin to note what frames of reference are used by the family members in discussing their difficulties. By *frames of reference* we mean whether there exists a family or an individual problem, which individuals seem to be bearing the brunt of the blame, how the identified problem members deal with their role, who has overt power in the family, what are the alliances in the family, who seems to get interrupted by whom, who speaks for whom, who seems fearful or troubled about expressing an opinion, who sits next to whom, and so forth.

The nonverbal communication of families is a key to family patterning. It is also often difficult to follow and interpret. Videotaping a family interaction is one way to closely observe nonverbal communication, which may be expressed by a child who twiddles his thumbs in the same way as his mother, a father whose facial expression and bodily movements indicate the opposite of what he is actually saying, or a parent who stares off into space when his adolescent son yells. All of these observations are as valuable as some of the verbal comments that the family may make to the interviewer.

Why Does the Family Come for Treatment at the Present Time?

The answer to the question of why the family has come for treatment at this time helps to shift the focus of difficulty closer to the current situation and also provides an opportunity for further specifying the kinds of factors that lead to family distress. The various types of last-straw situations usually present the important patterns of family interaction in a microcosm.

> In the B family, a son, C, age 25, has had symptoms of paranoid schizophrenia for many years. The parents allowed C to sleep in their bedroom at night. On the day after he moved out to his own apartment, Mr. and Mrs. B began to blame each other for the son's behavior and sought attention because their son was "out on the

streets, where anything could happen." The son had maintained an uneasy balance between the parents by staying in the parental bedroom at night, thus obviating their need for intimacy or sex. It was only when he moved out that the parents' problem came into sharp focus.

The answer to the question above also helps alert the therapist to any acute crisis situation that may need either the therapist's or the family's immediate intervention. The answer will be relevant, too, in assessing the goals the family has in mind for the therapy and the degree to which the family is motivated for help.

Until recently, it was usually the wife who requested psychotherapy for herself or brought the family, under protest. This most commonly reflects women's greater sense of responsibility for the family's emotional functioning and their willingness to accept blame or guilt and to seek and accept expert help, rather than their having a greater degree of intrapsychic disturbance. However, with the popularization of therapy, and family therapy in particular, over the last decades, men have become more attuned to family issues and more comfortable with therapy as a possible solution. The therapist must understand that there are usually very different levels of motivation in different family members, whether split on gender or other lines.

The therapist must be sure to determine the referral context and history. This includes referral source(s), conflict and agreement among family members or referral source(s), current involvement in other treatment (including medical), history of prior treatment (type, hospitalization, outcome, satisfaction), and the presence of other informal treaters.

What Is the Background of the Family Problem?

The therapist should obtain the following information:

1. *Composition and characteristics of the nuclear and expanded family, including age, sex, occupation, financial status (note differences between husband's and wife's income as well as*

joint financial status), medical problems, and so on. Race, class, and ethnicity are important data here. Couples from ethnic groups with widely differing traditions or communication styles often have problems in communication. If the couple has moved up or down a social class from the parent generation, this is important to note. A genogram (three-generation) can be used. This is a graph of the patient and several generations of the patient's family, noting important dates (births and deaths, marriages, separations, etc.), occupational role, and major life events such as illness. It also has symbols and conventions (Figure 4–1). A good example of a genogram is provided in Figure 4–2. For the sake of clarity, it is drawn without symbols (see "The Family Genogram" later in this chapter).

2. *Developmental history and patterns of each family member.* Individual family members' life histories are evaluated in terms of patterns of adaptation, including an impression of how the individual manages affects, frustration, and identity outside the family. Although somewhat outside the scope of a family therapy text, our bias is that the evaluator should not underestimate the importance of individual styles of adaptation, the use of defenses and resistances, tolerance of stress and ego strengths, signs and symptoms of any mental disorder, and the capacity of each person to be supportive and empathic to his or her partner.

3. *Developmental history and patterns of the nuclear family unit.* The longitudinal course of the family unit is explored with reference to the role of the spouses' individual expectations, values, goals, and conflicts in their relationship; the effect of each partner's adaptive patterns on the other partner; how gender roles have been expressed over time in the family; the need for control by one partner or the other, including how control is obtained and maintained; the existence of mutual trust and ability to share; the importance of individual and mutual dependence issues; and the family's ability to deal effectively with its earlier life phases (in the family's life cycle).

4. *Current family interactional patterns (internal and external).* Is the power structure flexible, rigid, or chaotic? Are the genera-

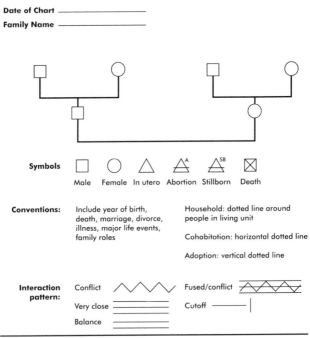

Date of Chart _____

Family Name _____

Symbols	□	○	△	△ᴬ	△ˢᴮ	⊠
	Male	Female	In utero	Abortion	Stillborn	Death

Conventions: Include year of birth, death, marriage, divorce, illness, major life events, family roles

Household: dotted line around people in living unit

Cohabitation: horizontal dotted line

Adoption: vertical dotted line

Interaction pattern: Conflict ∧∧∧ Fused/conflict

Very close Cutoff

Balance

FIGURE 4–1. **The family genogram and symbols.**
Source. Reprinted from Glick ID, Berman EM, Clarkin JF, et al: "The Content of Evaluation," in *Marital and Family Therapy,* 4th Edition, 2000, p. 160. Copyright 2000, American Psychiatric Press, Inc.

tion boundaries intact, blurred, or broken? Is there an affiliative or oppositional style? What degree of individuation is noted? Is there clarity of communication, tolerance for ambivalence and disagreement, respect for others' differences (as opposed to attempts at control or intrusiveness), responsiveness to others, and an ability to deal realistically with separation and loss? Do the family beliefs seem congruent to the situation? What is the overall family affect: that of warmth, humor, caring, hope, ten-

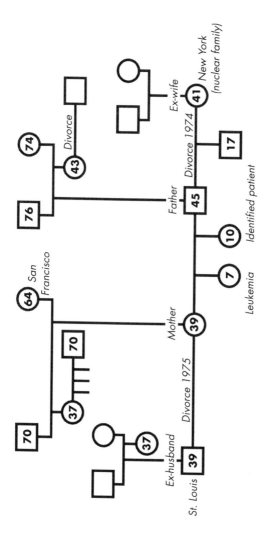

FIGURE 4–2. **Example of a genogram.**

derness, and the ability to tolerate open conflicts, or that of constricted, unpleasant, hostile, and depressive or resentful behavior?

This part of the evaluation—the background of the family problem—lends itself to expansion or contraction, depending on the circumstances. For example, a profound examination of a particular sector of the family's current functioning or past history might be thought relevant in a particular instance. In another situation, only a brief amount of background data might be gathered initially, with the feeling that more will emerge as the treatment sessions proceed. In any event, the therapist would always want to identify the important participants in the family's current interactions, the quality of the relationships, and the developmental patterns of the family unit over a period of time.

What Is the History of Past Treatment Attempts or Other Attempts at Problem Solving in the Family?

It usually is illuminating to understand the circumstances that led a marital couple or family to seek assistance in the past, from what sort of helpers this assistance was elicited, and the outcome of this assistance. Experience in previous help-seeking efforts serves to illuminate more clearly both the family processes and possible therapist traps and delineates useful strategies. Past help-seeking patterns are often useful predictors of what the present experience will be in both family therapy as well as other therapies.

The D family came into treatment presenting the complaint that they could not get along with each other and were contemplating divorce. They gave a history of being in family therapy several years before. They had had some 20 sessions, which "of course led to nothing." In discussion with the couple and the former therapist, it was discovered that the couple had spent most of the sessions blaming each other and attempting to change each other, rather than making any change in their relationship or in themselves. In addition, Mr. D, who was authoritarian, had persuaded the therapist to line up on his side and say that his wife was unreasonable. This treatment had been unsuccessful. The strategy in this case was to go over in detail the past problems in treatment and to suggest that the present therapist would not be a judge and that the focus was to be on the couple's relationship and on each partner's own responsibility for change in himself or herself, rather than on what the other partner would have to do.

Often one spouse has been in intensive individual psychotherapy to seek help with the marital relationship. When this has proven unsuccessful, both therapist and patient may blame the failure on the spouse not in treatment. This may exacerbate the difficulty and lead to separation or divorce.

Mrs. E began individual therapy because she felt her husband was inadequate. Her own life had been replete with difficulties, starting from the time she had lost both her parents in an automobile accident when she was 2 years old. She had lived in various orphanages, had been in two marriages by the time she was 22, and had periodic bouts of alcoholism and depression. She felt that her present marriage of 5 years had been "okay" until she had had children. She felt that, although she had had some difficulty in raising the children, the real problem was in her husband. She attended individual psychotherapy three times a week, and in the course of this began to "see quite clearly what a loser he was." Although her therapist struggled valiantly to point out her own difficulties at first, he too began to see the difficulties in the husband. The husband himself was never called into therapy, and after 2 years of treatment the couple was still experiencing the same problems and were contemplating divorce. A consultant suggested marital therapy.

What Are the Family's Goals and Expectations of the Treatment and Their Motivations and Resistances?

Some families come to treatment for short-term goals, such as finalizing a fairly well-thought-out separation between husband and wife. Others come for more long-term goals, such as making a basic change in how the family functions. Other families come because of an individual-oriented goal (the mother's depression), whereas still others come because of a family goal ("the family isn't functioning right"). In a case in which the goals are individual oriented, the therapist's task is to translate for the family the relationship between the symptoms and the family process. Initial goals will at times be unclear or unrealistic. In such instances the therapist and the family must work out from the beginning an appropriate, clear set of goals.

The marital couple and family presumably have certain types of positive hopes and motivations for seeking help but at the same time have some hesitations, doubts, and fears. One of the therapist's tasks is to explore and reinforce the positive motivations, to clarify them, and to keep them readily available throughout the process of therapy, which at times may be stormy and stressful. In marital therapy, the motivation of each partner for joint therapy should be evaluated. The evaluation should include the partners' stated commitment to the marriage, the evaluator's opinion of their commitment to therapy, the reality of their treatment expectations, and the opinions of other interested parties as related by the pair, such as those of parents or friends (and sometimes extramarital partners).

Positive expectations, goals, and motivations keep the family members in treatment, and every effort should be made to ensure that each family member benefits from the family therapy sessions as individuals and also as concerned members of the family. It is helpful to work out these expectations explicitly between family members and the therapist.

Ideally, it is desirable for each involved family member to clearly understand the positive reasons for his or her own participation, as well as the more general family system goals. At the same time, the therapist must be aware of individual and family resistance before it undermines either the successful use of treatment or its actual continuance. Clinical judgment will suggest when such fears and resistances need immediate attention and when they need to be only kept in mind as potentially major obstacles.

Such resistances may be of various sorts. Although some may be specific to particular families, many are general concerns. Among these is the feeling that the situation may be made worse by treatment; that some member of the family will become guilty, depressed, angry, or fearful as a result of the treatment; that a family member may go crazy; that the family may split up; that there is no hope for change and it is already too late for help; that shameful or damaging family secrets may have to be revealed; or that perhaps it would be better to stick to familiar patterns of family interaction, no matter how unsatisfying they may be, rather than attempt to change them in new and therefore frightening directions.

> In the F family, the wife felt that to continue in marital therapy after her recovery from an acute psychotic episode might mean that she would go crazy again. She believed that she and her husband would have to explore their unsatisfactory marriage and that this might lead to separation or divorce. She also felt that she would have to be strong and powerful to prevent her husband from committing suicide in the same way that his own father had committed suicide, presumably in relation to having a weak, unsupportive wife. The husband, for his part, had a very obsessional personality structure with little interpersonal sensitivity or emotional awareness. He felt angry at psychiatrists and was insecure and threatened by the therapist as a male role model. The evaluator with this couple would need to look for and stress the strengths of the couple and allow them to avoid discussing areas of maximal sensitivity before they were ready.

The family evaluation outline, Parts III and IV, as shown in Table 4–1, is discussed in Chapter 5.

■ THE FAMILY GENOGRAM

Even in the absence of a comprehensive assessment scheme such as our family evaluation outline (see Table 4–1), the family genogram remains an extremely popular tool for couples and family assessment. The genogram, developed by Bowen (1978), is a three-generational map of family relationships. Usually the genogram is developed during the beginning phases of a treatment and serves many process as well as content purposes:

1. It provides the patient, family, and therapist with a structure with which to explore current difficulties and their background.
2. It gives the therapist background information with which to put current difficulties in context.
3. The process of gathering the information may give the patient some conception, distance, and control over the emotional tugs and pulls created by the family.
4. It can be used later in the therapy to set realistic goals for dealing with the emotional strains of the family system in the future.

The genogram displays information about the family in a graphic, accessible fashion so that the therapist and family can begin to understand how present family circumstances may be linked to the family's evolving context of relationships. McGoldrick and Gerson (1985) have written the most comprehensive text on using the genogram. They provide a format for the standard genogram symbols and outline the principles underlying the effective application and interpretation of the genogram. In Figure 4–1, we have included the genogram form used in the Couples and Family Therapy Clinic at Stanford University Medical Center. Therapists routinely collect this information from the couple or family, often on a whiteboard, so that family members can observe its unfolding and make additional contributions. Clinicians then transcribe the data on the form shown in Figure 4–1 and include it in their clinical chart. Genograms should be a routine part of any assessment.

■ REFERENCES

American Psychiatric Association: Diagnostic and Statistical Manual of Mental Disorders, 4th Edition, Text Revision. Washington, DC, American Psychiatric Association, 2000

Bowen M: Family Therapy in Clinical Practice. New York, Jason Aronson, 1978

Emde RN: Clinical Psychiatry News, November 2001, p 9

Epstein NB, Bishop DS: Problem-centered systems therapy of the family, in Handbook of Family Therapy. Edited by Gurman S, Kniskern DP. New York, Brunner/Mazel, 1981, pp 444–482

Gill M, Newman R, Redlich F: The Initial Interview in Psychiatric Practice. New York, International Universities Press, 1954

Group for the Advancement of Psychiatry: The Case History in the Study of Family Process. Report No 76. New York, Group for the Advancement of Psychiatry, 1970

Haley J: Problem-Solving Therapy. San Francisco, CA, Jossey-Bass, 1976

McGoldrick M, Gerson R: Genograms in Family Assessment. New York, WW Norton, 1985

Minuchin S: Families and Family Therapy. Cambridge, MA, Harvard University Press, 1974

Napier A, Whitaker C: The Family Crucible. New York, Harper and Row, 1978

Reiss D: The Family's Construction of Reality. Cambridge, MA, Harvard University Press, 1981

5

FORMULATING AN UNDERSTANDING OF THE FAMILY PROBLEM AREAS

Meeting with the family, the therapist experiences its patterns of interaction and uses the data obtained to begin formulating a concept of the family problem. These formulations come from historical material and from the direct observations made during contact with the family. The data gathered should permit the therapist to pinpoint particular dimensions or aspects of the family functioning, and its individual members, that may require special attention. As data are gathered, the therapist notes areas of health and dysfunction and creates a priority list for addressing problems. Prioritizing a family's problems allows the therapist to focus on the relative severity of the issues, establishing which should be dealt with first and in what order. The data also enable the clinician to have greater clarity about therapeutic strategy and the tactics indicated for the particular phases and goals of treatment.

■ RATING IMPORTANT DIMENSIONS OF FAMILY FUNCTIONING

Using the explicit interview data, and drawing heavily from observation of the family in interaction during the evaluation sessions, the therapist is in a position to formally or informally summarize and rate the important dimensions of function.

Communication

In assessing a family's communication, the major focus is on the quality and quantity of information exchange among the family members. Can they state information clearly and accurately? Is that information listened to and perceived accurately by the other family members? Can some family members do this, whereas others cannot? Is the tone of the communication (the command aspect) respectful? Affirming? Demanding? Insulting?

Problem Solving

Every family is faced with problems. One difference between nondistressed and distressed families is that the latter do not come to effective agreement and action on problems, which then accumulate. The family has come for evaluation with at least one problem, and by asking about current and prior attempts at solving this problem, the interviewer gets a sense of where and how the family has started. Many authors (Jacobson and Christensen 1996) have delineated the steps of effective problem solving, and some have made teaching of these problem-solving steps a major ingredient of family intervention. In the assessment, it is important to note which of the steps in the problem-solving sequence the family is capable of: 1) stating the problem clearly and in behavioral terms, 2) formulating possible solutions, 3) evaluating the solutions, 4) deciding on one solution to try, and 5) assessing the effectiveness of that solution.

Roles and Coalitions

Basic tasks must be taken care of in the family unit, including the provision of food, clothing, shelter, money, nurturing and support, and sexual gratification of the marital partners. The notion of roles refers to the recurrent patterns of behavior by various individuals in the family through which these family tasks are carried out.

Furthermore, as the individuals in the family carry out their functions, how do they coordinate and mesh with others in the family? How rigidly are roles assigned by age or gender, rather than by ability? Who assumes leadership, especially around issues of decision making? To what extent does the family seem fragmented and disjointed, as though made up of isolated individuals? Or does it rather appear to be one relatively undifferentiated ego mass? How are boundaries maintained with respect to family of origin, extended family, neighbors, and community? To what extent is the marital coalition functional and successful? To what extent are there cross-generational dyadic coalitions that are stronger than the marital dyad? How successfully are power and leadership issues resolved?

Affective Responsiveness and Involvement

In looking at affective responsiveness and involvement, the clinician assesses the family's ability to generate and express an appropriate range of feelings. To what extent does the family appear to be emotionally dead rather than expressive, empathic, and spontaneous? What is the level of enjoyment, energy, humor? To what extent does there appear to be an emotional divorce between the marital partners? To what extent does the predominant family mood pattern seem to be one of depression, suspicion, envy, jealousy, withdrawal, anger, irritation, and frustration? To what extent is the family system skewed around the particular mood state or reaction pattern of one of its members? Are the emotions expressed consonant with the behaviors and context?

Affective involvement refers to the degree of emotional interest and investment the family members show with one another. This could range from absence of involvement through involvement that is devoid of positive feelings, narcissistic involvement, warmth and closeness, and angry intrusiveness, to symbiosis (L. Wynne, personal communication, November 1987).

Behavior Control

Behavior control is the pattern of behavior the family uses to handle physically dangerous situations (e.g., a child running into a road, reckless driving), expression of psychobiological needs and drives (e.g., eating, sleeping, sex, aggression), and interpersonal socializing behavior. Control in these areas can range from rigid to flexible to laissez-faire to chaotic.

The most important initial assessment and intervention involve the prevention of physical harm to the family members or to the therapist. Abused children, battered wives, and sometimes battered husbands, as well as abused grandparents, are all too common. Violence directed toward therapists is not uncommon. Neither the family nor the therapist can work on other issues when they are afraid.

Encouraging family members to call the police when threatened, to seek shelter when abused, and to inform the appropriate authorities of child abuse should be regarded as the beginning of family therapy and as necessary for its success. The therapist in some circumstances is required to call child protection services regardless of whether the family wants it.

Operative Family Beliefs and Stories

Families and individuals function with a set of ideas (conscious and unconscious) about "what our family is about," what the family's history tells about the roles of men and women, what values are important (money, education, endurance) and what adults and children should do and be. Some of these ideas are clearly cultural or class bound, such as whether family loyalty or career advancement are more important and whether obedience or initiative is valued more in children. Some are due to issues in the family's history, such as a history of occupational success or failure or a parent who was in a war or the Holocaust. Some beliefs are about a particular child, in terms of whether he or she is good, bad, talented, or pretty, labels with which others, outside the family, might disagree. Some ideas are about therapy itself and whether people should accept help, do it on their own, or deny and endure problems. These beliefs markedly influence how the family functions and copes. Not all family members share each belief.

Recent Family Events and Stresses

In answering the question of why a family comes for treatment at a particular time, the therapist should carefully review any recent changes in family composition (births, deaths, recent marriages), location (a child leaves home), or stress (severe illnesses) and life cycle transition points.

■ FAMILY CLASSIFICATION AND DIAGNOSIS

Several generations of family therapists have attempted to find a reliable and agreed-on way to classify family functioning. Such attempts usually use problem-focused descriptive diagnosis, as exemplified by relational problems listed in DSM-IV-TR (American Psychiatric Association 2000) (Table 5–1) and the more complete Committee on the Family of the Group for the Advancement of Psychiatry (GAP) Classification of Relational Disorders (CORD) (Guttman et al. 1996; Table 5–2). The conditions described in these systems are serious ones, such as family violence with abuse of children. They are called *relational* diagnoses in that they involve interactions of one or several of the participants. (It is important to remember, however, that not all families have a diagnosis.)

For the family therapist, several dimensions of the family are important—the location and type of the problem (e.g., a marital conflict, a parent-child conflict with violence); the severity of the identified problem; the severity of general family dysfunction; and the description of the problematic system, which includes both the history and the current patterns of communication, role, affect, and so forth. It is critical to determine whether the problem is heavily weighted toward issues of the individual (e.g., a child with schizophrenia in a reasonably well-functioning family) or toward issues of the family (e.g., a marital relational disorder with violence in the midst of a divorce).

Table 5–3 presents a schematic way of addressing key questions for the therapist. The task includes making a *diagnosis,* mean-

---

TABLE 5–1.   **DSM-IV-TR relational problems and problems related to abuse or neglect**

Relational Problems

Relational problems include patterns of interaction between or among members of a relational unit that are associated with clinically significant impairment in functioning, or symptoms among one or more members of the relational unit, or impairment in the functioning of the relational unit itself. The following relational problems are included because they are frequently a focus of clinical attention among individuals seen by health professionals. These problems may exacerbate or complicate the management of a mental disorder or general medical condition in one or more members of the relational unit, may be a result of a mental disorder or a general medical condition, may be independent of other conditions that are present, or can occur in the absence of any other condition. When these problems are the principal focus of clinical attention, they should be listed on Axis I. Otherwise, if they are present but not the principal focus of clinical attention, they may be listed on Axis IV. The relevant category is generally applied to all members of a relational unit who are being treated for the problem.

V61.9   Relational problem related to a mental disorder or general medical condition

This category should be used when the focus of clinical attention is a pattern of impaired interaction that is associated with a mental disorder or a general medical condition in a family member.

V61.20   Parent-child relational problem

This category should be used when the focus of clinical attention is a pattern of interaction between parent and child (e.g., impaired communication, overprotection, inadequate discipline) that is associated with clinically significant impairment in individual or family functioning or the development of clinically significant symptoms in parent or child.

V61.10   Partner relational problem

This category should be used when the focus of clinical attention is a pattern of interaction between spouses or partners characterized by negative communication (e.g., criticisms), distorted communication (e.g., unrealistic expectations), or noncommunication (e.g., withdrawal) that is associated with clinically significant impairment in individual or family functioning or the development of symptoms in one or both partners.

TABLE 5–1.   **DSM-IV-TR relational problems and problems
related to abuse or neglect** *(continued)*

V61.8   Sibling relational problem

This category should be used when the focus of clinical attention is a
pattern of interaction among siblings that is associated with clinically
significant impairment in individual or family functioning or the
development of symptoms in one or more of the siblings.

V62.81   Relational problem not otherwise specified

This category should be used when the focus of clinical attention is on
relational problems that are not classifiable by any of the specific
problems listed above (e.g., difficulties with co-workers).

Problems Related to Abuse or Neglect

This section includes categories that should be used when the focus of
clinical attention is severe mistreatment of one individual by another
through physical abuse, sexual abuse, or child neglect. These problems
are included because they are frequently a focus of clinical attention
among individuals seen by health professionals. The appropriate V code
applies if the focus of attention is on the perpetrator of the abuse or
neglect or on the relational unit in which it occurs. If the individual being
evaluated or treated is the victim of the abuse or neglect, code 995.52,
995.53, or 995.54 for a child or 995.81 or 995.83 for an adult (depending
on the type of abuse).

V61.21   Physical abuse of child

This category should be used when the focus of clinical attention is
physical abuse of a child.

Coding note: Specify 995.54 if focus of clinical attention is on the victim.

V61.21   Sexual abuse of child

This category should be used when the focus of clinical attention is sexual
abuse of a child.

Coding note: Specify 995.53 if focus of clinical attention is on the victim.

V61.21   Neglect of child

This category should be used when the focus of clinical attention is child
neglect.

Coding note: Specify 995.52 if focus of clinical attention is on the victim.

TABLE 5–1.   **DSM-IV-TR relational problems and problems related to abuse or neglect** *(continued)*

Physical abuse of adult

This category should be used when the focus of clinical attention is physical abuse of an adult (e.g., spouse beating, abuse of elderly parent).

Coding note: Code

V61.12 if focus of clinical attention is on the perpetrator and abuse is by partner

V62.83 if focus of clinical attention is on the perpetrator and abuse is by person other than partner

995.81 if focus of clinical attention is on the victim

Sexual abuse of adult

This category should be used when the focus of clinical attention is sexual abuse of an adult (e.g., sexual coercion, rape).

Coding note: Code

V61.12 if focus of clinical attention is on the perpetrator and abuse is by partner

V62.83 if focus of clinical attention is on the perpetrator and abuse is by person other than partner

995.83 if focus of clinical attention is on the victim

Source.   Reprinted from American Psychiatric Association: *Diagnostic and Statistical Manual of Mental Disorders,* 4th Edition, Text Revision. Washington, DC, American Psychiatric Association, 2000, pp. 736–739. Copyright 2000, American Psychiatric Association. Used with permission.

ing both a systemic and a dynamic formulation. Both formulations are done for both the individual and the family. The questions are:

- How can the problem best be explained (boxes A, B, C, D)?
- What is the level of family functioning, and how does the family function—that is, what are the family problems and processes (box C)?
- Do one or more family members have a DSM-IV-TR Axis I, II, or III diagnosis (box D)?
- If there is a serious psychiatric disease in one or more family members (box D), how is the family involved (box A)?

TABLE 5–2.   **Proposed classification of relational disorders**

I.   Relational disorders within one generation

   A.   Severe relational disorders in couples

      1.   Conflictual disorder with and without physical aggression

      2.   Sexual dysfunction

      3.   Sexual abuse

      4.   Divorce dysfunction

      5.   Induced psychotic disorder (folie à deux)

   B.   Severe relational disorders in siblings

      1.   Conflictual disorder

      2.   Physical and/or sexual abuse

      3.   Induced psychotic disorder (folie à deux)

II.   Intergenerational relational disorders

   A.   Problems relating to infants, children, and adolescents

      1.   With overt physical abuse or neglect

         a.   With intrafamily child sexual abuse

         b.   Without sexual abuse

      2.   With problems in engagement

         a.   Overinvolvement

            i.   Intrusive overinvolvement

            ii.   Emotional abuse

            iii. Family separation disorder

               (a)   Preadolescent type

               (b)   Adolescent type

          b.   Underinvolvement

            i.   Reactive attachment disorder

            ii.   Failure to thrive

      3.   With problems in control

         a.   Undercontrol

         b.   Overcontrol

         c.   Inconsistent control

      4.   With problems in communication

         a.   Communication deviance (for example, high expressed emotion)

         b.   With lack of affective or instrumental communication

TABLE 5–2. **Proposed classification of relational disorders** *(continued)*

B. Problems relating to adult offspring and their parents
    1. With physical abuse or neglect
    2. With problems in engagement
        a. With burden
        b. With overinvolvement
    3. With problems in communication
        a. With cutoffs
        b. With severe verbal conflict

Source. Reprinted from Guttman HA, Beavers WR, Berman E, et al: "A Model for the Classification and Diagnosis of Relational Disorders." *Psychiatric Services* 46:926–931, 1995. Used with permission.

TABLE 5–3. **A comprehensive evaluation schema**

Type of formulation	For the family	For the individual(s)
Functional diagnosis	**A** A systemic formulation	**B** Behavioral or individual psychodynamic model and/or biological model
Descriptive diagnosis	**C** DSM-IV-TR conditions not attributable to a mental disorder that are a focus of attention or treatment (e.g., parent-child problem, family typology)	**D** DSM-IV-TR classification for each family member on Axis I, II, or III, as appropriate

Source. Adapted from Glick ID, Berman EM, Clarkin JF, et al: *Marital and Family Therapy,* 4th Edition. Washington, DC, American Psychiatric Press, Inc., 2000, p. 176. Copyright 2000, American Psychiatric Press, Inc. Used with permission.

- How can systems concepts help in understanding the problem (box A)? What are the roles of individual biology (box B) and individual psychodynamics (box B) in understanding the problem?

Finally, the therapist can determine the severity of the family problem, using the Global Assessment of Relational Functioning (GARF) (Table 5–4). This is a dimensional scale (e.g., communication is a dimension) that describes features of a relationship along a continuum from health to dysfunction. It permits the clinician to characterize the overall functioning of a family or other ongoing relational unit on a hypothetical continuum from competent, optimal performance to disorganized, maladaptive functioning. The GARF scale includes only three areas of family functioning: problem solving, organization, and emotional climate. As a global scale, GARF cannot characterize all of the features of families and other relationships that might be important to specialists assessing and treating families, but it is still very useful.

Approaching it another way, the therapist can

- Use the DSM-IV-TR or the GAP diagnostic scheme for a descriptive diagnosis, if applicable
- Describe the functioning of the family, using the dimensions listed earlier in this chapter
- Make a judgment as to the salience of individual pathology
- Determine the severity of the family problem, using GARF

■ PLANNING THE THERAPEUTIC APPROACH AND ESTABLISHING THE TREATMENT CONTRACT

After the evaluation data have been gathered and formulated into diagnostic hypotheses, goals regarding important problem areas can be formulated. The therapist is then ready to consider what therapeutic strategies will be appropriate.

TABLE 5–4. **Global assessment of relational functioning (GARF) scale**

Instructions: The GARF scale can be used to indicate an overall judgment of the functioning of a family or other ongoing relationship on a hypothetical continuum ranging from competent, optimal relational functioning to a disrupted, dysfunctional relationship. It is analogous to Axis V (Global Assessment of Functioning Scale) provided for individuals in DSM-IV. The GARF scale permits the clinician to rate the degree to which a family or other ongoing relational unit meets the affective or instrumental needs of its members in the following areas:

A. *Problem solving*—Skills in negotiating goals, rules, and routines; adaptability to stress; communication skills; ability to resolve conflict

B. *Organization*—Maintenance of interpersonal roles and subsystem boundaries; hierarchical functioning; coalitions and distribution of power, control, and responsibility

C. *Emotional climate*—Tone and range of feelings; quality of caring, empathy, involvement, and attachment/commitment; sharing of values; mutual affective responsiveness, respect, and regard; quality of sexual functioning

In most instances, the GARF scale should be used to rate functioning during the current period (i.e., the level of relational functioning at the time of the evaluation). In some settings, the GARF scale may also be used to rate functioning for other time periods (i.e., the highest level of relational functioning for at least a few months during the past year).

Note: Use specific, intermediate codes when possible, for example, 45, 68, 72. If detailed information is not adequate to make specific ratings, use midpoints of the five ranges, that is, 90, 70, 50, 30, or 10.

81–100   Overall: *Relational unit is functioning satisfactorily from self-report of participants and from perspectives of observers.*

Agreed-on patterns or routines exist that help meet the usual needs of each family/couple member; there is flexibility for change in response to unusual demands or events; and occasional conflicts and stressful transitions are resolved through problem-solving communication and negotiation.

TABLE 5–4. **Global assessment of relational functioning (GARF) scale** *(continued)*

There is a shared understanding and agreement about roles and appropriate tasks, decision making is established for each functional area, and there is recognition of the unique characteristics and merit of each subsystem (e.g., parents/spouses, siblings, and individuals).

There is a situationally appropriate, optimistic atmosphere in the family; a wide range of feelings is freely expressed and managed within the family; and there is a general atmosphere of warmth, caring, and sharing of values among all family members. Sexual relations of adult members are satisfactory.

61–80 Overall: *Functioning of relational unit is somewhat unsatisfactory. Over a period of time, many but not all difficulties are resolved without complaints.*

Daily routines are present, but there is some pain and difficulty in responding to the unusual. Some conflicts remain unresolved but do not disrupt family functioning.

Decision making is usually competent, but efforts at control of one another quite often are greater than necessary or are ineffective. Individuals and relationships are clearly demarcated, but sometimes a specific subsystem is depreciated or scapegoated.

A range of feeling is expressed, but instances of emotional blocking or tension are evident. Warmth and caring are present but are marred by a family member's irritability and frustrations. Sexual activity of adult members may be reduced or problematic.

41–60 Overall: *Relational unit has occasional times of satisfying and competent functioning together, but clearly dysfunctional, unsatisfying relationships tend to predominate.*

Communication is frequently inhibited by unresolved conflicts that often interfere with daily routines; there is significant difficulty in adapting to family stress and transitional change.

Decision making is only intermittently competent and effective; either excessive rigidity or significant lack of structure is evident at these times. Individual needs are quite often submerged by a partner or coalition.

Pain or ineffective anger or emotional deadness interferes with family enjoyment. Although there is some warmth and support for members, it is usually unequally distributed. Troublesome sexual difficulties between adults are often present.

TABLE 5–4. **Global assessment of relational functioning (GARF) scale** *(continued)*

21–40 Overall: *Relational unit is obviously and seriously dysfunctional; forms and time periods of satisfactory relating are rare.*

Family/couple routines do not meet the needs of members; they are grimly adhered to or blithely ignored. Life cycle changes, such as departures or entries into the relational unit, generate painful conflict and obviously frustrating failures of problem solving.

Decision making is tyrannical or quite ineffective. The unique characteristics of individuals are unappreciated or ignored by either rigid or confusingly fluid coalitions.

There are infrequent periods of enjoyment of life together; frequent distancing or open hostility reflects significant conflicts that remain unresolved and quite painful. Sexual dysfunction among adult members is commonplace.

1–20 Overall: *Relational unit has become too dysfunctional to retain continuity of contact and attachment.*

Family/couple routines are negligible (e.g., no mealtime, sleeping, or waking schedule); family members often do not know where others are or when they will be in or out; there is little effective communication among family members.

Family/couple members are not organized in such a way that personal or generational responsibilities are recognized. Boundaries of relational unit as a whole and subsystems cannot be identified or agreed on. Family members are physically endangered or injured or sexually attacked.

Despair and cynicism are pervasive; there is little attention to the emotional needs of others; there is almost no sense of attachment, commitment, or concern about one another's welfare.

0 Inadequate information.

At this point, a beginning contract with regard to goals and treatment should be established (Shankar and Menon 1993). This should include who is to be present; the location, times, estimated length, and frequency of meetings; and the fee and contingency planning with respect to absent members and missed appointments. Some therapists contract for 10 sessions and renew, whereas others leave things open ended. For some families, treatment will be very brief and crisis oriented, lasting only one or two sessions, whereas for other families, treatment may continue for months or, in some cases, years.

The therapist should then make a concise, explicit statement of the family problem, using language the family can understand. The treatment model the therapist is using will determine such a formulation. For example, a behavioral therapist might explain that "You two have gotten into the habit of criticizing each other so much that you have neglected to comment on the good things the other one does, or to give each other what each of you needs. We will try to help you to communicate more clearly and to take care of each other in ways that you each want." A more dynamic approach might be "Each of you had a mother who was depressed and a father who was working too hard to be available. So each of you assumes that if the other one doesn't give you what you want, the other one must be unavailable or unloving. It makes both of you become tense and withdrawn a lot. Perhaps we can find a way to help you separate your past from your present and learn to take care of each other better." A problem-solving approach might be "You seem to be trying to explain to each other what you need in ways that make each of you angry. So your attempts to solve this problem have been making things worse. Per haps we could find a better way to do it, by focusing on the solutions that have worked at least some of the time."

Some therapists may want to refer families to a book specifically written for the lay market, entitled *Solving Your Problems Together: Family Therapy for the Whole Family* (Annunziata et al. 1996). Clinical examples can be found in *Marital and Family Therapy,* 4th Edition (Glick et al. 2000).

■ MEDICAL EXAMINATIONS

To rule out physical problems as the cause of individual or family dysfunction, medical examinations may need to be completed for each family member when indicated. Major psychiatric illness should be evaluated by using traditional history-taking and mental-status examinations. Physical illness must also be kept in mind.

■ HOME VISITS

In some instances, a family therapist might choose to visit the family in its own home, with as many family members present as possible. Sometimes the reason may be that a critical family member is disabled or housebound. At other times, home visits can be considered when the therapist senses a gross discrepancy between the interactions observed in the office sessions and the reports of what is taking place at home.

Home visits enable the therapist to see the family on its own turf and may lead to a better understanding of its interactional patterns. Some families have the feeling that the therapist is more interested when he or she is willing to make a home visit. However, there are possible disadvantages to home visits. For example, the family may see the visit as an intrusion or may try to convert the therapy into a purely social situation. In general, the rationale and timing of the visit can vary depending on its purpose, but it should always be discussed with the family and agreed to in advance.

■ FAMILY TASKS

Assessment techniques in which the entire family is involved in a structured task have also been developed. For example, if the therapist recommends that the family plan a picnic together or furnish a room together (using hypothetical furniture and a fixed amount of money), he or she can observe their problem-solving processes, coalitions among family members, roles, and areas of conflict. Such techniques give the family therapist useful ways of evaluating families in which verbal interventions are not the common communication method. Therapists should continually look for ways to assess and intervene in the couple's or the family's process by suggesting activities such as discussing a difficult issue, watching the process unfold, and supporting what is functional while gently challenging what is not. These local experiments provide the therapist with in vivo data that are very useful because they represent a behavior sample that most closely approximates the family's behavior outside the session.

Therapists can also assign tasks or homework in between sessions to assess the couple's or the family's motivation, flexibility, and resourcefulness. For example, asking a very intellectualizing family to go bowling together may provide them with an alternative form of enjoying each other while letting the therapist learn about their willingness to engage in novel behaviors. Tasks can be playful (e.g., "Each time one of you remembers to compliment the other, you get a penny"). They can also be very serious, as when the therapist asks parents to track the antecedents and consequences of problem behaviors shown by their school-age child over the week.

For the clinician who wants a view of the actual ecology of the family, meal time is notable as a microcosm of the family in sociological and dynamic terms. The therapist can make direct observations of family meal planning, preparation, and consumption. Alternatively, the family therapist can ask the family to describe the seating and behavior at a typical family meal. Sometimes family members will not eat together. Children rather than parents may prepare the meals. An adolescent who is angry with his or her parents will often take meals alone, if the parents allow this. One particular child might be used as a mediator between the parents and may be asked to sit between them, whereas the other siblings are not so involved in the parental drama. In a situation in which one parent cannot function (for example, a drinking father), that parent may take meals in the bedroom. Such observations are often helpful in determining the family patterns. Either in session or between sessions, family tasks are a rich source of clinical data.

■ REFERENCES

American Psychiatric Association: Diagnostic and Statistical Manual of Mental Disorders, 4th Edition, Text Revision. Washington, DC, American Psychiatric Association, 2000

Annunziata J, Annunziata J: Solving Your Problems Together: Family Therapy for the Whole Family. Washington, DC, American Psychological Association, 1996

Glick ID, Berman EM, Clarkin JF, et al: Marital and Family Therapy, 4th Edition. Washington, DC, American Psychiatric Press, 2000

Guttman HA, Beavers WR, Berman E, et al: A model for the classification and diagnosis of relational disorders. Journal of Psychiatric Services 46:926–932, 1995

Guttman HA, Beavers WR, Berman E, et al: Global Assessment of Relational Functioning scale (GARF), I: background and rationale. Group for the Advancement of Psychiatry Committee on the Family. Fam Process 35:155–172, 1996

Jacobson N, Christensen A: Integrative Couple Therapy. New York, Norton, 1996

Shankar R, Menon MS: Development of a framework of interventions with families in the management of schizophrenia. Psychosocial Rehabilitation Journal 16:75–91, 1993

6

GOALS IN FAMILY TREATMENT

■ MEDIATING AND FINAL GOALS AS THEY RELATE TO SCHOOLS

One convenient way to conceptualize types of treatment goals is to distinguish *final goals* (the ultimate results desired) from the *mediating (or intermediate) goals* that must precede the final results. Although one would conceptualize unique and specific goals for each individual family, more general mediating (Table 6–1) and final (Table 6–2) family therapy goals are presented here. These are relatively broad areas that allow for considerable flexibility according to the specifics of each particular family or marital unit, and they are not mutually exclusive but often intertwined.

The problems of families and the goals specific to them, both mediating and final, should determine the strategies of the therapy.

■ INDIVIDUALIZING GOALS WITH THE FAMILY

The therapist forms a concept of the family's difficulties based on an evaluation of the family's history and interaction. The treatment often begins with the issues that seem to be most crucial to the family; the treatment at the outset helps the family to deal with an immediate crisis situation. Only after some stability and rapport have been achieved is it possible for the therapist to begin to help the family in areas that will also be beneficial. The work is sometimes slow and gradual, but often a few sessions are enough to get the family's own adaptive mechanisms operating again. At most family

TABLE 6–1.   **The most common mediating goals**

1. *Establishment of a working alliance.*   Patients and families size up therapists very quickly, and these early attitudes are likely to persist. Thus, the early connection between the family therapist and each family member is crucial to the ultimate outcome of the work. Setting up such an alliance in individual therapy seems relatively simple in comparison with setting up an alliance with the multiple members of a family, who themselves often do not get along with each other. The therapist also must find a way to connect with each person rather than favoring certain family members.

2. *Specification of problem(s).*   Specifying problems includes a detailed delineation of family members' feelings and behaviors around the symptoms or problems that brought the family to treatment.

3. *Clarification of attempted solutions.*   Many families have attempted solutions to their problems before concluding that they need outside intervention. Because almost invariably these solutions have failed, the therapist should determine what did not work (as, indeed, some would say that many problems are simply ordinary situations to which poor solutions were applied).

4. *Clarification and specification of individual desires and needs.*   Each family member's desires and needs must be clarified and specified as they are expressed, mediated, and met in the total family/marital environment and network of relationships. It is the lack of clarity and conflict (either overt or covert) around such needs and desires that leads to or constitutes family pathology itself.

5. *Modification of individual expectations or needs.*   The therapist must help each family member to understand that individuals can change only so much, but that even small individual changes can produce profound family changes. Over the course of treatment, members of the family may modify their expectations. Greater appreciation of the family's contributions may occur, as well as increased reliance on oneself or sources outside the family.

TABLE 6–1.   **The most common mediating goals** *(continued)*

---

6. *Recognition of mutual contributions to the problem(s).*   Therapists differ in how much they think recognition of family members' mutual contributions to problems must come early in the therapy or how explicit it must be. However, the very acceptance of the family intervention format (most or all family members coming to most sessions) implies some recognition of mutual contribution to the problem or at least to solutions.

7. *Redefinition of the problem(s).*   Redefining a problem completely or redefining it into various parts, some of which are problematic and others not, are all steps to possible solutions. By way of an example, the therapist might say, "You are not bad people; you are responding to stress with anxiety or anger."

8. *Improvement of communication skills.*   Communication skills include listening and expressive skills, diminution of coercive and blaming behavior with an increase in reciprocity, and effective problem-solving and conflict resolution behaviors.

9. *Shifting disturbed, inflexible roles and coalitions.*   Changing roles and coalitions may include helping to improve the autonomy and individualization of family members, fostering the more flexible assumption of leadership by any particular family member as circumstances require, and facilitating general task performance by one or more members.

10. *Increasing family knowledge about psychiatric illness.*   In families that have one or more members with serious Axis I pathology, such as schizophrenia or recurrent affective illness, a common mediating goal is to increase family information about the illness, its course, and its responsiveness to environmental, including familial, stresses.

11. *Fostering insight into historical factors related to current problems or into current interaction patterns.*   This mediating goal may be relatively important in psychodynamically oriented family or marital work and may be absent in other orientations. However, other orientations may reframe particular stories about the family's history as a way of changing interactions.

TABLE 6–2. **The most common final goals**

1. Reduction or elimination of symptoms or symptomatic behavior in one or more family members[a]
2. Resolution of the problem(s) as originally presented by the family
3. Increased family/marital intimacy
4. Role flexibility and adaptability within the family matrix
5. Toleration of differentness and differentiation appropriate to age and development level
6. Balance of power within the marital dyad and appropriate sharing of input and autonomy for the children
7. Increased self-esteem
8. Clear, efficient, and satisfying communication
9. Resolution of neurotic conflict, inappropriate projective identification, and marital transference phenomena

[a]These symptoms may include major or minor symptoms of mood and affect (anxiety and depression), thought disorder, disruptive behaviors in children and adolescents, marital conflict and fighting, and sexual disorders.

therapy clinics, the average number of visits is 6–10. One hallmark of family therapy is the belief that rapid change is possible. Sometimes a family comes in for a brief period for one problem and returns later to work on additional issues. Consistent with current attitudes in medicine and other helping professions, family therapists do not consider this a failure. When one member is seriously ill, therapy may be long term, intermittent, and supportive.

In setting goals, it is helpful to think not only of the family as a whole and of the various interpersonal dyads and triads but also of the individuals who make up the system. Each individual has a history, a personality, and a set of coping mechanisms. A thorough knowledge of individual personality theory and psychopathology is essential for knowing what to expect from the individual "atoms" as well as from the family "molecule." At times it will be necessary to provide specific treatment for, or to direct specific attention to, the needs of an individual family member (for example, when a family member is floridly psychotic) with individual sessions, somatic treatment, and sometimes hospitalization.

Even under ordinary circumstances, however, a thorough understanding of the strengths and weaknesses of each family member (basic personality patterns, reactions to stress, and so on) will help to determine the goals and techniques of family therapy. Especially when separation or divorce impends, it becomes critical to assess individual issues.

In setting goals, it is also important to assess the needs of the larger family system, that is, those who may be deeply involved in the family but not in the room. For example, if the wife's mother hates her son-in-law and wishes her daughter would divorce, this is a critical issue affecting the nuclear family. In addition, the possibilities within the larger social system must be considered. For example, is it possible for a couple to marry if it means losing a significant amount of money from public assistance or alimony?

The goals of family treatment must be congruent in some way with what the family members seem to desire and what they are realistically capable of achieving at any particular point. The therapist's views of the appropriate therapeutic possibilities, however, may differ from those initially envisioned by the family members. For example, the family may wish for a home with no conflict, whereas the therapist might see a need for more effective ways of disagreeing.

Overall goals encompass the entire family system as well as its individual members. Ideally, the entire family should function more satisfactorily as a result of family therapy, and each family member should derive personal benefit from the experience and results of the therapy. The family therapist, for example, should not be in the position of taking the focus off a scapegoated member (saying, for instance, "It's not Dad's withdrawal that is the problem") only to consistently refocus on one or another family member as the cause of the family's difficulties. Nor should the family as a whole feel blamed for one member's problems.

Some families today seek professional help not for these more traditional reasons, however, but rather for clarification of family roles and as a growth-enhancing experience. Of course, this is less common because of managed care, unless the family self-pays for the therapy. In such cases, a problem-solving model seems less appropriate than a growth-development model.

■ GOALS AND THEIR RELATION TO PROCESS AND CONTENT ISSUES

The relative importance of structure and process, as compared with content, is an issue sometimes raised by family therapists. The more traditional view tends to favor substantive content issues, whereas the newer, holistic view looks more closely at the characteristic patterning in an interpersonal network, placing less emphasis on the subject matter. In some ways this may be an artificial dichotomy. For example, the communication process may become the most important subject matter of the therapy. Any attempt to deal with a specific content issue inevitably brings process issues to the surface (and vice versa).

> The G family requested help because their 19-year-old son, H, was very angry at his mother and was living at home but was verbally abusive and refused to help the household in any way. The problems started when H was supposed to go to college but refused. In sessions, which included H, his mother, his father, and his younger brother, H would talk angrily and dominate the sessions, while his mother would complain about him whenever he stopped talking. H's father and his younger brother watched silently. An initial goal was to alter the communication pattern to bring the rest of the family into the session and decrease the intensity between the mother and H. The content of what the mother and H talked about was less relevant than the context and pattern of the communication. The therapeutic interventions were to insist that H make room for the other members of the family, to get the father to support the mother, and to connect the sibling subsystem. Only when the communication pattern was altered did it become clear that H had stayed at home both out of fear of failure (he had always had some trouble at school, and college would be a big step) and because he was afraid that his father's diabetes would worsen and he would be needed at home.

■ MEDIATING GOALS AND THEIR RELATED STRATEGIES

The art of psychotherapy is by definition the intersection of appropriate mediating goals with the most efficient therapeutic strategies and techniques at the most propitious moment and in the right sequence. The various ways of conceptualizing overall strategies of family intervention are summarized in Table 6–3.

TABLE 6–3. **Goals and strategies common to family therapy schools**

---

1. *Supporting adaptive mechanisms.* There are a number of ways to help families to use existing strategies and to develop new strategies for coping. Examples include providing the family with information (psychoeducation) about illnesses in family members and about parenting skills and giving supportive advice and encouragement of existing coping mechanisms. A related strategy is "bearing witness"—acknowledging and understanding the family's experience or emotional pain or trauma, both of which are of critical importance.

2. *Expanding emotional experience.* Basic skills are listening, labeling, and encouraging supportive family response to feeling. Sharing the therapist's own response or that of others (e.g., saying "Many people would feel great pain in that situation") is a main way of validating and encouraging feeling. Therapists may at times use fantasy, humor and irony, direct confrontation, family sculpting, and choreography to open up new areas of immediate emotional experiencing for the family.

3. *Developing interpersonal skills.* By a multitude of techniques, including modeling of intent listening to others, insisting that only one person speak at a time, questioning the exact meaning of what others are saying and wishing to communicate, and explicit instruction in communication skills, the family is brought to a better communication level. This improvement in communication levels can be an end in itself or can be used to solve specific problems that initially brought the family to treatment.

TABLE 6–3. Goals and strategies common to family therapy schools *(continued)*

4. *Reorganizing the family structure.* Reframing problems as presented by the family, enacting the family problems with their attendant interactional sequences, marking boundaries, and restructuring moves can all be used to change the structured family behaviors that are judged to be causing or contributing to family distress. Paradoxical interventions, although less used now, can be used for families that are resistant or at an impasse.

5. *Increasing insight.* Traditional techniques of psychodynamic psychotherapy, such as clarification, confrontation, and interpretation—regarding either recent dynamic issues or old, repetitive family interactional patterns of long duration—can be used in marital and family treatment formats. Such techniques can bring underlying conflicts to the fore and reduce conflict-laden interactions. Insight here must be relational, in terms of how the person's past affects the present and the response of the other. Another useful way of developing insight is direct questioning of the parents and analysis of current relationships through family-of-origin work.

6. *Helping the family understand and modify its narrative.* These strategies involve helping the family tell their story and find alternative and less problem-saturated narratives that offer novel solutions. Both the therapist and family members look for redefinitions (enthusiastic rather than noisy, survivor rather than victim), understandings (fear of failure rather than laziness), and novel outcomes (what about the times it doesn't fail—what happens then?).

7

FAMILY TREATMENT: STRATEGIES AND TECHNIQUES

Before describing how to treat families, we must first examine family therapy in the general context of the strategies and techniques of psychotherapy. In this chapter, the recommended treatment modalities extend beyond the notion that success is merely an unconditional acceptance of life and what it brings. Subjective and objective improvement should be seen in behaviors, emotions, and individuals' capacities to live.

Each of the various strategies for treating families emphasizes different assumptions and types of interventions. Some therapists prefer to operate with one strategy in most cases, whereas others combine these strategies depending on the type of case and the phase of treatment. At times the type of strategy used is made explicit by the therapist, whereas in other instances it remains covert; however, irrespective of whether a therapist specializes in one or another approach or is eclectic, some hypotheses will be formed about the nature of the family's difficulty and the preferable approach to adopt.

Therapists may choose one school or another on the basis of their training or their personality. Individuals and families may also prefer some ways of working over others. This text encourages the integration of a variety of techniques depending on the particular problem and personalities of the family. It also encourages the therapist to look beyond the problem at hand, that is, the presenting complaint, to issues of power, intimacy, and personal growth. Our approach is to emphasize models based on empirical data.

■ GENERAL ELEMENTS OF PSYCHOTHERAPY AND THEIR RELATIONSHIP TO FAMILY THERAPY

Most schools of psychotherapy commonly share a number of elements:

- An effective patient-therapist relationship
- Release of emotional tension or development of emotional expression
- Cognitive learning
- Insight into the genesis of one's problems
- Operant reconditioning of the patient toward more adaptive behavior patterns, using techniques such as behavioral desensitization
- Suggestion and persuasion
- Identification with the therapist
- Repeated reality testing or practicing of new adaptive techniques in the context of implicit or explicit emotional therapeutic support
- Constructing a more positive narrative about oneself and the world
- Instilling hope

Family therapy, too, involves all of these elements, but does so in the context of the whole family and has as its goal the improvement of the overall functioning of the entire group. The particular mix of therapeutic elements varies with the specific needs of the family. There is hardly any specific technique used in other therapy formats (individual and group) and orientations (psychodynamic, cognitive-behavioral, strategic, experiential-humanistic) that could not in some way be adapted for use in family intervention.

■ BASIC STRATEGIES OF FAMILY INTERVENTION

Because there is much overlap in the schools of family intervention (both in theory and techniques), and because it is our bias that the field must advance beyond narrow schools to basic principles of change, we present here our choice of the basic strategies of family intervention. We also provide a description of the techniques used in each of these strategies. Basic to family therapy are strategies for the following:

- Supporting adaptive mechanisms, supporting and encouraging strengths, and imparting new information, advice, and suggestions (psychoeducational approach)
- Expanding individual and family emotional experience
- Explicit development of interpersonal skills, such as communication skills, parenting skills, and problem-solving skills
- Reorganizing the family structure
- Increasing insight and fostering intrapsychic conflict resolution
- Helping the family find new and more positive ways of understanding their situation (narrative approach)

These strategies, abstractly stated in terms of their aims or goals in treatment, are not mutually exclusive. To some extent, they represent different frames of reference for understanding and dealing with the same family phenomena. Nevertheless, each strategy offers something unique in its conceptualization and execution. The choice of strategy depends on the goals, but in general all families can benefit from a review and support of their strengths.

In a clinical situation, the therapist will be hard put to remain a purist. A therapist's efforts to clarify communication may produce shifts in family coalitions or may initiate an exploration of family myths that may lead to a considerable outpouring of previously concealed affect.

Although some specific therapeutic strategies are listed here, no one magical phrase or technique will cure the family. Interventions are instead a series of repetitive maneuvers designed to change feelings, attitudes, and behaviors. If the overall goals and strategy are kept in mind, specific interventions will suggest themselves and will be modified by the particular circumstances and the therapist's own style. What is unique in family therapy is not so much the specific technique used but the fact that these techniques are used not with an isolated individual but within a relationship, and that the overall focus and strategy aim to evaluate and produce a beneficial change in the entire family system.

Techniques for Supporting Adaptive Mechanisms

First and foremost, the therapist uses many techniques to support the active or latent positive coping mechanisms that the family has at its disposal. Every family has some health, and this should be acknowledged and actively encouraged. Empathic listening and concern, positive feedback about the use of adaptive defenses (such as healthy denial in the face of a fatal illness) and education about poorly adaptive defenses, and well-timed advice are all helpful to the family in distress.

The therapist is constantly in the role of a teacher, either directly or indirectly. Without saying a word, he or she models mood, tempo, and interpersonal acceptance. The therapist also teaches values, often implicitly. For example, in structuring the treatment so that only one person in the family speaks at once, the therapist models good communication but also implicitly reinforces the value of respecting the thoughts of every person in the family.

Recently there has been a growing emphasis on providing explicit information that might be helpful to families in their coping. This approach has been most obvious in the psychoeducational strategies used in families with a member with a diagnosed disorder such as schizophrenia (Anderson et al. 1986; Goldstein 1996). Information can be communicated through written material, lectures and discussions in family groups, and in workshop format. Anderson et al. (1986) describe a day-long survival skills workshop that the family attends without the patient. Information is provided on the nature of schizophrenia (its history and epidemiology, biology, personal experience), medication and psychosocial treatments, and the role of the family (family reactions to the patient and the illness, coping with the condition).

> Ms. I was a 20-year-old, white, single female college student with long-standing double depression (i.e., major depressive disorder and atypical depression) since her early teens. She was in the midst of an 8-month episode of acute depression characterized by psychomotor retardation, cognitive slowing, lability, and overeating. She was being treated with a combination of individual therapy, family therapy, and antidepressants. Although she had been ill for 3 or 4 years, she had never understood her illness. Her physician spent time explaining in detail the multiple roots of her depression. She reported that before receiving the psychoeducation, when she thought about her illness it was "like a huge something I don't understand." After psychoeducation, she stated that she could "pick apart pieces of the illness and ask questions about it and understand it, and I felt better immediately after the session." When pressed as to why she felt better, she said her thoughts were more cohesive and thus she could better cope with her illness.

A second nuance of psychoeducation involves the family therapist's focus on the patient's perception that she was lazy because she spent so much time on the couch watching television. The intervention directed to the patient and the family was partly psychoeducational (i.e., it was explained that "leaden paralysis" is a cardinal symptom of atypical depression and weight gain is a side effect of antidepressants) and partly dynamic and systemic.

The educational approach need not be limited to situations in which there is a clear diagnosis of a condition whose etiology has biological components. Communication skills and problem-solving skills are taught in many forms of marital therapy. For example, Patterson (1982) provides information to parents with antisocial children so that they can improve their family management skills. Likewise, in some situations, there are families who function relatively well, to whom the therapist gives advice. This may include discussing parenting alternatives (such as discipline styles) or helping the family to make difficult decisions (e.g., whether a child should go away to school or stay at home).

The use of psychoeducation should not lead to either biological or behavioral reductionism. As Hunter et al. (1988) have pointed out, "family therapists should not abandon a concern with the inner lives of severely ill patients and their families after they are educated about an illness." Families asked about their experience in therapy repeatedly cite as helpful the therapist's ability to listen respectfully, to notice their strengths, and to actively offer suggestions and advice in a respectful and not a commanding manner. Families need to have the sense that their therapist has ideas they can try, but that the therapist will not be hurt or angry if they do not agree with the plan.

Techniques for Expanding Emotional Experience

Techniques used to help individuals and family units expand their experience repertoire tend to focus on the here-and-now experience in the sessions themselves. These techniques are designed to help the individual family members to quell anxiety, slow down their reaction process, and maximize the emotional and cognitive experience of the moment—experiences that may have been denied, defended against, and missed in the past. In many families, feelings are either avoided or detoured. For example, some members of the family, or the entire family, may not admit to feelings because they are afraid of hurting another member. Alternatively, certain feelings may be avoided or denied, so that, for example, anger may be expressed instead of sadness. Rebellious or inappropriate behavior may be used as a nonverbal protest (forgetting, daydreaming, or encopresis as a way of demonstrating helpless rage or anxiety). In some families the affect, especially rage or anxiety, may appear all too obvious and overwhelming, but invariably there are hidden feelings as well, and silent family members. Some families may appear too full of affect, whereas some families may seem to have none. The therapist's job is to slow down or speed up the family's process and allow the variety of feelings to surface in a safe environment, allowing everyone to feel heard and to see how hidden or detoured feelings or long-standing rage or anxiety have affected the family's functioning. It is important to understand that in families often the most important thing is to know that other people understand how one feels, even when they cannot fix it. For a child especially, the most difficult thing, even worse than disagreement or punishment, is to be disconfirmed—that is, to feel completely ignored.

The therapist's main role is to look for the likely feelings and help the family members to express them, using empathy and clarification. Simple examples of such expression are: "That really must have hurt"; "How did you feel then?"; "I hear that you were angry, but you also look sad; why is that?" The therapist may also use disclosure, such as "That story makes me feel sad." This is especially helpful in younger patients who are less experienced in expressing strong emotions that are often felt by the child to be overwhelming. The therapist then asks how other family members felt or reacted, because the issue in families is not only the feeling but also the reaction or anticipated reaction of other family members. "Did you tell your Mom or your Dad how you felt? What did they say? How did you feel, Mom? Dad? What happened next? Were there other people in the family who felt differently? Why? If you didn't tell them then, how do you think they feel when you tell them now?" The therapist acts as witness and support, making sure that everyone is heard and also protected. The therapist looks at which feelings are and are not acceptable in the family and whether only certain family members express things for others (e.g., only the mother expresses anxiety and is told she is crazy).

This technique is particularly important in marital therapy, where the spouses' feelings about each other form much of the basis of the therapy. The sense that one is not heard or respected by another is a common underlying reason for divorce in a society that, as we have said, has assigned the fulfillment of emotional needs as the center of marriage. Ensuring that both partners feel heard is critical when there is violence, acting out, or mourning. When the feelings are of great grief or there is great anger and a need to forgive, often rituals are designed to support or accentuate the process. For example, families that have been unable to mourn may be asked to prepare a new memorial service, to share stories and perhaps pictures of the deceased with the therapist, or to design a new holiday celebration that would include memories of the person who died but allow for new activities. A number of techniques adapted from other therapies are also powerful emotional catalysts, including psychodrama and the techniques adapted from it—role play, gestalt and family sculpting, family marathons, and guided fantasy. Although these are all interesting and often extremely powerful techniques, they are best left to those with special training. In the long run, there are few forces as powerful as a therapist who can sit with a family, hour after hour, in the face of their pain, bearing it with them and helping them find ways to heal.

Techniques for Developing Interpersonal Skills

Many families and marital units do not use basic skills of communication, parenting, and general problem solving. This may be either because they have never learned such skills due to poor or absent parental modeling or because of interpersonal conflicts that interfere with the use of such skills.

The therapist is by training an expert in communication and thus can help family members express their thoughts and feelings more clearly to one another. These are not skills traditionally learned in residency and are not always the property of beginning therapists. The therapist should be certain that he or she is familiar with these techniques and should have attempted to use them on a personal level before teaching them to others. The therapist tries to promote open and clear communication, emotional empathy, and a positive rapport between family members, as well as good problem-solving skills. Good problem solving requires an additional set of skills beyond the clear communication of feeling. Communication requires both a speaker and a listener (or a communicator and a receiver, in the case of nonverbal communication) and consists of not only the message sent, but also the message intended and the message received. The goal of the therapist is to help the family to look at intended messages, the way in which the message is sent and its content, and what the receiver thought about it. Although it is impossible not to communicate in a family (silence plus nonverbal signals is a powerful message), nevertheless, many troubled family members spend very little time talking meaningfully with one another. Not only thoughts but also feelings are distorted, hidden, negated, or blurred. The person sending the message may or may not be aware that his or her intention and the message do not match, and unless the person asks, he or she will never know what the other person understood.

The therapist supplies an arena for family discussion, being cognizant of the different levels of meaning in messages and how these influence and sometimes contradict each other. The therapist does not allow anyone to monopolize a session or to speak for someone else. The therapist helps the family to look at how messages are sent, what messages are hidden, and why it is often difficult to hear them. One common technique to slow down a conversation so that it is clearer is to insist that, before someone can reply to a communication, he or she has to repeat it back, first verbatim and then in paraphrase:

Example of problem:
Husband: I was really upset that you didn't do the dishes last night.
Wife: You think I'm a bad wife and mother! Well, you didn't do the breakfast dishes either.
Example of communication practice:
Husband: I was really upset that you didn't do the dishes last night.
Wife: You were really upset that I didn't do the dishes.
Husband: Yes, that's what I said.
Wife: That makes me angry! And I think you think I'm a sloppy person.
Husband: I don't think you are sloppy, but you promised to do them. I am upset because you broke your promise to me, and that makes me feel as if you don't care about me.

The therapist attempts to encourage interpersonal sensitivity and empathy and tries to help each person become more aware of his or her own thoughts and feelings.

The therapist encourages family members to be specific, to state who did what to whom (for example, "Dad hit me with a stick" rather than "He did it"). The therapist encourages more productive and supportive communication. He or she emphasizes finding positive as well as negative ways of saying things and noticing nonverbal messages. With children, the therapist helps the parents speak to the child in ways that are appropriate to the child's age. The therapist looks for people who speak for others (e.g., a mother who always answers for her daughter) and for people who don't speak to each other (e.g., a son who never speaks to his mother but only to his father) and works to get people to speak for themselves ("I" statements) and to have people who have issues with each other speak directly to each other rather than through a third person. The therapist stresses that individuals are held accountable for their actions. He or she fills in gaps in communication, points out discrepancies, and deals with nonverbal communication. The therapist points out nonproductive verbal and nonverbal family communication patterns and tries to identify the implicit, unstated patterns or attitudes that may be causing trouble. Through these efforts, the covert is made overt; the implicit is made explicit. Blocked channels of communication and feeling can be opened up. The therapist counsels that good communication includes listening. Often three or four family members are heard talking at exactly the same time during a session, presumably to avoid hearing thoughts and feelings other than their own. The therapist in such a situation may function as a communications traffic cop or referee.

Marital and family life is filled with problems, large and small. Problem solving is different from sharing feelings in that the emphasis is on cognitively finding solutions to problems rather than simply expressing feelings about them. *Although expressing one's feelings may involve great positive or negative affect, problem solving requires calmness.* In many cases, distressed families have no more problems than nondistressed families have, but nondistressed families use effective problem-solving techniques so that problems are handled and do not multiply. Distressed families can be taught problem-solving methods. The steps of problem solving are 1) defining a problem, 2) brainstorming, 3) negotiating, and 4) making clear the behavioral contract. *In general, distressed families have problems with this process not only because of skill deficits but also because of hidden agendas,* many of which involve hidden power issues. For example, if a wife wants her husband to share more of the housework and he doesn't want to, a behavioral contract about how many nights he is to wash dishes is not likely to be of much help. The husband is likely to forget, to do the job badly, and to be angry, even if the wife agrees to do something for him in return. The problem must be defined as a larger issue about equality in family life, and if the husband is strongly against doing any more work, it is difficult to solve. It will have to be clear to him that he will get something of equal value that will not injure his sense of self-esteem or manliness (the cognitive issue behind the behavioral problem). A couple or family who comes up with seemingly reasonable solutions that are not put into practice needs to spend time with the therapist in redefining the problem and looking for the issues behind the issues.

In addition to the communication and problem-solving skills needed by a marital dyad, additional skills are needed to raise children effectively. Patterson (1982) has referred to these as family management skills and has devised techniques for teaching these skills to families with an antisocial child. The family management skills that can be taught include rule setting, parental monitoring (detection and labeling), and parental sanctions, including the appropriate use of positive reinforcement and punishment. Each of these skills must be carefully taught, role-played, and supervised.

In the social learning theory tradition, Stuart (1980) has outlined a behaviorally oriented marital therapy package that begins with assessment and proceeds through caring days (i.e., each partner in a couple offering specifically requested caring behaviors; increasing small, high-frequency, conflict-free behaviors; communication skills; contracting procedures; training in problem-solving skills; training in conflict containment; and strategies for maintaining the changed interaction). He gives as a clinical example a "holistic agreement," in which several behaviors by one spouse are exchanged for several by the other, with no requirements that the offerings by one exactly match those of the other. For example, an agreement arrived at by J and K, negotiated and put in writing, looks like the following. J would like K to share in washing the dishes, mow the lawn, initiate lovemaking, and take responsibility for balancing their checkbooks. K would like J to have dinner ready by 6:30 nightly, weed the rose garden, and call K at the office daily. It is contracted and expected that each will do as many of the things requested by the other as is comfortably manageable, ideally at least three or four times weekly. This model is workable only if the therapist has carefully looked at the power, intimacy, and justice issues underlying the problematic behaviors. Most behaviorally oriented marital therapies stress cognitive issues (e.g., How does this fit with my picture of myself? Is this acceptable behavior in my culture?) as well as carefully and gradually increasing the positive and caring behaviors. Systemic and cognitive approaches are gradually joining (see Dattilio et al. 1998).

Strategies and Techniques for Changing Structured Family Behaviors

In many ways, the unique contribution of the family orientation is the recognition of structured (repetitive and predictable) behavioral sequences in family groups that contribute to the etiology and/or maintenance of symptomatic behaviors. A "typical" four-member family is taken as the unit (Figure 7–1).

In example A in Figure 7–1, the functional family, the marital coalition is the strongest dyad in the family, the generation boundary is intact, and all other channels are open and about equal in importance to one another. In contrast to this are the various types of dysfunctional families that follow.

In example B, the marital coalition is relatively weak or absent, and instead there are strong alliances across the generations and the sexes—between father and daughter, mother and son—and a rela-

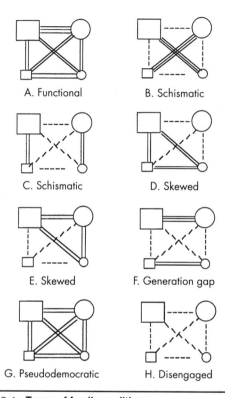

A. Functional

B. Schismatic

C. Schismatic

D. Skewed

E. Skewed

F. Generation gap

G. Pseudodemocratic

H. Disengaged

FIGURE 7–1. **Types of family coalitions.**

Squares represent males; circles, females. Larger symbols stand for spouses/parents; smaller symbols, offspring/siblings. The solid straight lines joining these symbols represent positive communication, emotional, and activity bonds between the individuals involved, in a semiquantitative fashion, according to the number of straight lines used. Dotted lines represent the relative absence or negative quality of the interactions.

Source. Reprinted from Glick ID, Berman EM, Clarkin JF, et al: *Marital and Family Therapy,* 4th Edition. Washington, DC, American Psychiatric Press, 2000, p. 251. Copyright 2000, American Psychiatric Press. Used with permission.

tive absence of other effective channels. In example C, there are cross-generational alliances between same-sex parents and children. Examples B and C can be thought of as representing types of the schismatic family.

Examples D and E depict skewed families in which one family member is relatively isolated from the other three, who form a fairly cohesive unit. Example F represents the generation-gap family, in which the marital unit and the offspring each form a fairly cohesive duo with little or no interaction across the generation lines. Example G represents the pseudodemocratic family, in which all channels seem to be of about equal importance, with the marital coalition and the parental role not being particularly well differentiated. Example H, the disengaged family, represents an extreme case in which each family member is cut off from every other member, and in which one would expect very little sense of positive interaction, feeling, or belonging to a family unit.

Clearly these representations are highly oversimplified and are pictured only for a two-generation, four-member family. Infinite variations could be added to the list. Such representations enable the therapist to conceptualize more clearly the nature of the coalitions in a particular family and to begin planning a strategy to bring those coalitions into a better functional alignment, presumably more closely approximating example A. In example B, for instance, the therapist might give attention to activating the marital coalition, the coalitions between parent and offspring of the same sex, and those between the offspring themselves. Also, an attempt might be made to attenuate the force of the existing cross-generational, cross-sexed interactions.

The tactics and strategies of family therapy, viewed in this light, might include changes in the marital coalition (very commonly the case) as well as in the parent-child dyads. Although triads are not considered to any great extent in this model, an isolated family member might be brought into interaction with the rest of the family unit. In some of these families, the problem is an overly connected triad, in which case decreasing the less-functional coalitions will automatically make space for the isolate. Looking outside of the nuclear family for a moment, it is critical to consider coalitions and cutoffs with the extended family (e.g., parents and siblings of the adults, other significant family members) and to examine relationships with other significant systems (e.g., children's peers, therapists, or other helping professionals in the system, as well as secret relationships such as partners in extramarital affairs). Remarried families in particular have immensely complicated structures, and it is critical to use a genogram to include all members of the family. When such outside interactions, especially with in-laws, seem problematic, modifications should be considered. Sometimes outside interactions may need to be encouraged, especially in cases where no one has contacts outside the family.

Temporary triads incorporating the therapist are often purposely formed to produce structural change:

> In the L family, the father is primarily connected with his son, both men are disrespectful to the mother and the daughter, and the daughter enters therapy with depression. Rather than treat the daughter's depression in isolation, the therapist looks at how the father's disrespect and the mother's passivity have made her feel hopeless. The therapist encourages the husband to insist on his son being respectful (fathers teach their sons respect) and works with the parents to encourage the mother to speak up for herself and the father to look at why he is treating his wife badly. (For example, perhaps he is actually angry because she is paying attention to her mother and not to him.) The parents are encouraged to support their daughter and to deal with their own issues. The daughter's depression lifts because she no longer has to be her mother's support.

Techniques that enable the family therapist to interrupt and change such structured family behaviors are central to this understanding (Minuchin 1974; Minuchin and Fishman 1981). The techniques include those shown in Table 7–1.

Techniques for Insight and Conflict Resolution

Although experiential and psychodynamic schools of psychotherapy have different goals, both have in common the use of tech-

TABLE 7–1. **Family treatment techniques**

1. *Reframing:* Each individual *frames* reality from his or her own unique perspective. When the therapist perceives and understands the patient's or the family's frame and counters this frame with another, competing view, this is called a reframe (Watzlawick et al. 1974).

2. *Enactment:* It is one thing for a family to describe what has happened, and it is another thing for them to enact it in front of the therapist. Enactment is the technique of eliciting the playing out of interpersonal problems the family complains of in the therapeutic hour.

3. *Focusing:* The family therapist is flooded with a multitude of data from the patients. Treatment requires organization, highlighting, and progression in the treatment, and the therapist must focus the attention of the group. From multiple inputs, the therapist must select a focus and develop a theme for the family therapy work (Minuchin and Fishman 1981).

4. *Boundary making:* Boundary-making techniques are ways of focusing on and changing the psychological distance between two or more family members. The therapist can make boundaries by verbal reconstructions, giving tasks, special rearrangements of seating in the sessions, nonverbal gestures, and eye contact (Minuchin and Fishman 1981).

5. *Unbalancing:* The family therapist uses unbalancing techniques to change the hierarchical relationship of members of a family system or subsystem. There are three basic ways of unbalancing the existing family hierarchy and power distribution: 1) affiliating with certain family members, 2) ignoring family members, or 3) entering into a coalition with some family members against others. Unbalancing may have unintended consequences and should be undertaken with a clear sense of the reason for its use and with watchfulness to ensure that this intervention is working.

6. *Creating a systemic reality:* By use of mainly cognitive interventions, the family therapist attempts to help the individuals in the family perceive and understand the workings of their mutual interdependence and membership in an entity (the family) that is larger than themselves. Members of a family generally perceive themselves as acting and reacting to one another, rather than seeing the larger picture of the family "dance" over time.

TABLE 7–1.   **Family treatment techniques** *(continued)*

7. *Paradoxical techniques:*   These techniques are called "paradoxical"
    because they appear to be opposite to common sense. They are based
    on the fact that, although people are often aware of the reasons they
    want to change, it is the hidden reasons for not changing that keep the
    symptom going. Faced with a symptom that does not respond to
    support, insight, or logic, the therapist may suggest that the person
    keep the symptom to study its effects, make a list of all the reasons the
    symptom is useful or cannot be changed, or increase the symptom
    frequency to ensure that it is working (thereby proving that it is also
    under the person's control). Because it seems manipulative, many
    people have argued about this type of intervention. Most therapists
    reserve this type of intervention for more resistant couples (Weeks
    and L'Abate 1982).

---

niques to further the emotional-cognitive horizons of patients, with
the assumption that such expansion will lead to changes in behavior
and/or character. In expressive dynamic therapy, the therapist uses
the context of relative therapeutic neutrality (as well as empathic
support) to employ techniques such as clarification, confrontation,
and interpretation, either with the individual or the marital dyad or
family unit.

In family therapy, insight is always given in a family context.
In general, family therapists often feel that insight is more constructed than revealed. The goal is to link past with present reality
of the family in such a way that family members can stop trying to
solve the past with the present (Table 7–2).

Interpretations can be made in here-and-now interactions
between family members or between therapist and family mem-
ber(s), or interpretations can link present behavior to past history.
The former are probably of more use in family intervention. Ackerman (1958) was a pioneer in using dynamic techniques (along with
a multitude of others) in a family therapy format in order to interrupt intrapsychic conflicts being played out in the interpersonal
sphere.

TABLE 7–2. **Techniques for increasing insight**

---

1. *Clarification:*   In using the technique of clarification, the therapist asks the family to elucidate their understanding and/or emotional reactions to present and past events.

2. *Confrontation:*   Confrontation is the pointing out of contradictory aspects of the patient's behavior, often between verbal and nonverbal behavior.

3. *Interpretation:*   Interpretation is the elucidation by the therapist of links between present contradictory behavior and present or past distortions that are out of the awareness of the patient. In making interpretations, often immediately preceded by clarification and confrontations, the therapist provides a conceptual link for patient and family. It should be timed so as to maximize cognitive and emotional impact, between current behavior (as distorted or guided by internal templates) and past experiences (distorted by anxiety and defense mechanisms).

A couple in their 30s, married with three children, entered therapy complaining that the wife was not interested in sex. Although she was very busy with three young children, this did not seem to be the central issue. It was noted that the husband was very depressed and critical and had had serious depressive symptoms for years. He was treated with fluoxetine (Prozac) with excellent results. As his irritability lessened, the wife realized that she responded to his annoyance with fear and anxiety far beyond the usual response. At that point she began to discuss her abusive father and how if she made him angry he would hit her, or go into a total rage, and how desperately she had tried to be good. She was projecting onto her husband her fears about her father. The husband's mother had been intrusive and anxious, and when his mother became anxious his father would retreat, as the husband was doing with his own wife. As each recognized their projections, they began to learn to reassure the other, and the wife was able to relax and have satisfactory sex.

It is important to realize in this case that the issue was not oedipal (repressed sexual feelings toward the father) but the projection of an old family interaction into the present.

Dicks (1967), more than any other author, spelled out the use of dynamic techniques in the intervention with marital couples. Dicks describes a brief marital therapy case, quoted in the following:

H, a 45-year-old man, [was] married 20 years to W. The couple had three adolescent children. The presenting complaint was H's sexual impotence of 10 years' duration, depressive moods, and irritability, especially at his wife and children, all of which threatened his marriage.

In the initial diagnostic interview with H alone, he was asked about his early sexual attitudes. His associations shifted to his parental home and its atmosphere, noting that his sulking did not work as it did for his father, because he knows it is wrong. This was followed by an interpretation by the therapist: there seemed to be a similarity between general sulking and sexual withdrawal. The patient's next association was to his wife, whom he saw as having her own way as to times for intercourse. He then described the many talents of the wife in contrast to himself. Another interpretation was offered: You feel inadequate in comparison to W, as if she has all the potency, much as it was in your parents' case.

In the diagnostic interview with W, she described a strong bond to an idealized father who died when she was 17, and a scarcely concealed hostility toward a weak mother.

In the first conjoint marital session, it appeared that the couple had a stereotyped and unvarying pattern of attempting intercourse while simultaneously anticipating failure, followed by some symptomatic behavior on the part of the wife. In the second conjoint session, W suggested that they discontinue sleeping together, as the strain left her without sleep and constantly tired. An interpretation was made: her symptoms showed her emotional frustration, which might reflect her disappointment that H was not the strong, potent man she expected. She had tried to improve him, and H had met this with anxiety and resistance. H conceded that he left his office cheerful, but when he entered the home he felt depressed, nagged, and belittled. W responded by saying that it was not she but the children who got the brunt of his moods. She described her husband's belittling and sarcasm toward the children. Another dyadic interpretation was given: There is a vicious circle around power and control. H feels W is trying to control him, while he is feeling a great need to control the family through the children. W becomes anxious and resentful because she would like to run things her way. This battle has invaded their relationship, and the struggle to contain the urges to dominate has produced mutual strain and pushed out affection. The wife responded to this interpretation by conceding that she is driven to control, and sees how H responds by becoming controlling with the children. At this point the therapist suggested that this pattern may relate to earlier experiences in their families of origin. W recalled that she felt a lack of support from her mother and a devotion to her prematurely deceased father, a need to support and control the weak mother, and a desire that in marrying H he would make up for it all. An interpretation was made that she must feel very complicated about H's sexual difficulty and his feelings as the weak one. She now saw him not as the interested, inspiring father for her children in whom she saw her own needs mirrored. This interpretation was followed by a show of great feeling on the part of W, in which she recalled that the father was not only loving, but had also been very demanding and sarcastic, the latter so intolerable to her in H's behavior toward their children. Another interpretation: Perhaps W had not seen the similarity before between her feelings for H and for her father, with great disappointment that like her father H had weaknesses that she must control because she could not bear them. H responded with some emotion about how as a child he had been very strong willed and strove to compel his mother to give in to him. This was followed by a final dyadic interpretation: it was the strong-willed part of H that W liked. Because of his fear of weakness, the failure in sex, which could have happened to anyone under the circumstances, when it did, was quite disproportionately seen by H as an utter failure, with a compensatory need to control in the home. W, attaching her aspirations for strength and success on him, felt disproportionately disappointed in him because it destroyed her fantasy that he was like her father. Her reaction to disappointment, both in the past and now, was to take control.

By the third session, the couple reported that their general relationship was much improved, and the husband had been completely potent on a number of occasions.

Techniques for Finding New and More Positive Ways of Understanding the Family's Situation: The Narrative Approach

Among the newer additions to the field of family therapy is a set of assumptions falling loosely under the rubric of *constructivism,* part of the postmodern movement in philosophy and psychology. It is based on the work of a series of theorists from epistemology, biology, and cybernetics who see reality as constructed by the observer rather than a truth to be discovered. Translated into the field of therapy, this suggests that the family's reality is in its shared narratives and meaning systems, that the personal story or self-narrative provides the principal frame of intelligibility for our lived experience, and that the therapist's assumptions about the family are also constructed rather than being truth. The job of the therapist, then, is to help the family explore and reevaluate its own assumptions, beliefs, and meaning systems. In this model, a dysfunctional family has constructed a series of meanings that are not working in allowing the family flexibility and functioning. For example, if the mother is defined as bad, any move she makes toward either comforting or discipline will be ignored, meaning that the children get neither comfort nor discipline. If her story is constructed differently by the family, for example, as "Mother is doing her best to function despite her difficulties," she will be able to take care of the family, since they will accept her care. This model allows therapist and patient together to deconstruct confining family stories that produce stasis or sadness and to consider new ones. Rather than the therapist producing a reframed story and convincing the family of its correctness, this model emphasizes the importance of collaboration and mutual respect in the therapeutic alliance. Treatment is primarily conceptualized as a conversation about problems in which new meanings and new behaviors can be considered. Unlike those schools that highlight the family's history or its structural organization, these approaches highlight the strengths and competencies of the family that are often occluded by the family's and the therapist's tendency to focus on the problems that bring the family to treatment.

■ TREATMENT PACKAGES

Clinical work and research suggest that so-called treatment packages, which contain a combination of techniques delivered in some specified sequential fashion, are effective with targeted patient populations. These treatment packages include the prescribed use of various techniques from the major strategies described previously. Many of these packages include manuals that add to an abstract listing of strategies and techniques by indicating the overall goals, both mediating and final, of the treatment for the targeted families and provide a rationale for the timing and sequencing of the techniques of intervention. The field of psychotherapy research in general is in an era of research investigation of treatment packages (that is, the combination of a series of defined intervention techniques delivered in some prescribed order), as they are applied to specified disorders.

■ INDICATIONS FOR DIFFERENTIAL USE OF THE BASIC STRATEGIES

It is no wonder that trainees always ask when to use the various strategies and techniques differentially. This is an unresolved area, not only in the field of family therapy, but in all of psychotherapy. In their clinical zeal for their own favorite set of strategies and techniques, clinical writers usually do not discuss when their techniques are indicated and when they are not. Clinical research that has pitted one set of therapy techniques against another indicates that, by and large, no one technique is clearly superior. It remains for future research to clarify the differential application and effectiveness of the various techniques. However, in the interim, clinical decisions about the thrust of strategies in family intervention must be made on every case and in every session.

To choose a strategy, the therapist must consider both motivation and family style. Families who enjoy talking and analyzing, for example, may prefer a dynamic model, whereas action-oriented families may want specific homework and a behavioral model. Many, if not most, families want some educational interventions—

families want and need information. In addition, one must consider speed—less motivated families need something more quickly, so that brief therapy techniques are often the first techniques to try. Many apparently less-motivated families increase their motivation when they see results and begin to trust the therapist. One should also always remember the basic rule: try the simplest thing first. This is usually an explanation of the problem and some simple suggestion for making it better. Before one goes into an elaborate discussion of why a couple has become more distant, it is helpful to prescribe 15 minutes of talking to each other every night and see what happens. Sometimes this is all that is needed—if not, the therapist will get a lot of information from seeing how the couple avoided or sabotaged the task.

It is clear that some strategies of family therapy have received research support for their effectiveness, whereas others have been the focus of very little, if any, research.

Patient diagnostic issues are for the first time beginning to be important for recommended types of family therapy techniques. Patients with Axis I pathology, such as schizophrenia and bipolar disorder, and their families should receive psychoeducation about the illness and how to cope with it. It has also been argued that, because an individual with schizophrenia is, by the nature of the disorder, vulnerable to cognitive and emotional overload (which seems to be more true of males than females), family therapy strategies that stir up family emotional conflict should not be used, at least during certain phases of the disorder (Heinrichs and Carpenter 1983).

What the family wants is also very important. Most critical, however, is the family's sense that they are heard, understood, and respected and that the therapist believes that the problem can be solved, or at least made more tolerable.

It remains to be seen whether family classification schemes and typologies can be useful in guiding not only whether to use the family therapy format but also which strategies and techniques should be used in the family treatment format.

Because most of the therapy research has substantiated little differential effect for the various treatment strategies and techniques, some have argued that elements common to the various strategies are most important (Hoberman and Lewinsohn 1985). This would include careful assessment, focus as negotiated by the therapist, a reasonable rationale for proceeding, the generation of hope that intervention will help, and orientation to a goal. From this point of view, the organized approach of the family therapist is more important than the specific strategies and techniques. One clinical application of this notion is that the family therapist should not be eclectic in strategies to the point of shifting constantly from one set of strategies to another. A clear focus on the central family problems with a combination of a limited set of strategies is probably more efficient, less confusing to the family, and more effective. This is congruent with the fact that negative outcomes in family therapy are associated with a lack of therapist structuring and guiding of early sessions and the use of frontal confrontations of highly affective material early in treatment (Gurman and Kniskern 1978).

■ BEYOND TECHNIQUES

It has been wisely noted that a therapist, not unlike an artist, spends years of hard practice acquiring and honing techniques. Once acquired, these techniques become relatively invisible (Friedman 1974). During the 20 years before the turn of the millennium, family therapy saw a great deal of outcome research, from which manuals have been written. "The manuals attempt to carefully describe treatments, and therapists are taught to perform as the manuals describe. And, yet, with this careful attention to scientific rigor, researchers have noted that the same technique in the hands of a 'pro' and a 'neophyte' (despite years of practice) can have quite different effects on the patients" (M. Weissman, personal communication, February 1980).

■ REFERENCES

Ackerman N: The Psychodynamics of Family Life. New York, Basic Books, 1958

Anderson C, Reiss D, Hogarty G: Schizophrenia and the Family. New York, Guilford, 1986

Datillio F, Epstein N, Baucom D: An introduction to cognitive-behavioral therapy with couples and families, in Case Studies in Couple and Family Therapy. Edited by Dattilio F. New York, Guilford, 1988, pp 1–37

Dicks HV: Marital Tensions. London, Routledge and Kegan Paul, 1967

Friedman PH: Outline (alphabet) of 26 techniques of family and marital therapy: A through Z. Psychotherapy: Theory, Research and Practice 11:259–264, 1974

Goldstein MJ: Psychoeducation and family treatment related to the phase of a psychotic disorder. Int Clin Psychopharmacol 11:77–83, 1996

Gurman AS, Kniskern DP: Deterioration in marital and family therapy: empirical, clinical and conceptual issues. Fam Process 17:3–20, 1978

Heinrichs D, Carpenter W: The coordination of family therapy with other treatment modalities for schizophrenia, in Family Therapy in Schizophrenia. Edited by McFarlane W. New York, Guilford, 1983, pp 267–287

Hoberman HM, Lewinsohn PM: The behavioral treatment of depression, in Handbook of Depression: Treatment, Assessment and Research. Edited by Beckman EE, Leber WR. Homewood, IL, Dorsey Press, 1985, pp 39–81

Hunter DE, Hoffnung RJ, Ferholt BF: Family therapy and trouble: psychoeducation as solution and as problem. Fam Process 27:327–338, 1988

Minuchin S: Families and Family Therapy. Cambridge, MA, Harvard University Press, 1974

Minuchin S, Fishman HC: Family Therapy Techniques. Cambridge, MA, Harvard University Press, 1981

Patterson GR: Coercive Family Process. Eugene, OR, Castalia Publishing Company, 1982

Stuart RB: Helping Couples Change: A Social Learning Approach to Marital Therapy. New York, Guilford, 1980

Watzlawick P, Weakland J, Fisch R: Change: Principles of Problem Formation and Problem Resolution. New York, WW Norton, 1974

Weeks G, L'Abate L: Paradoxical Psychotherapy, Theory and Technique. New York, Brunner/Mazel, 1982

8

THE COURSE OF
FAMILY THERAPY

Without exception, trainees want and, in our opinion, need to review an entire course of treatment of a family, rather than experiencing only a one-session consultation or brief excerpts of a treatment. In this chapter, we review the stages of a typical course of treatment, somewhat arbitrarily dividing them into early phase, middle phase, and termination phase.

■ STRATEGIES FOR GETTING STARTED

Before describing in detail the specific techniques that enable the therapist to achieve the final goals of family intervention, it is important to note the general strategies used in beginning work with the family. These skills are basic, assumed by all orientations, and crucial for the neophyte to master. Without such skills, family dropout is likely, precluding any further possibility of change.

1. *Accommodating to and joining the family:*   The family is a biological-psychological unit that over time has evolved set rules (overt and covert), procedures, and customary interactional patterns. The therapist must come in from the cold and join this group by letting them know that he or she understands them and wants to work with and for their better good. Every family therapist will use his or her own unique personality, combined with sensitivity and warmth, to join with the family in distress.

2. *Interviewing various subgroups, extended family, and other networks:* Family therapy is by definition a therapeutic approach that emphasizes the tremendous power and influence of the social environment on the individual. This social environment includes the immediate family, the family of origin, the extended family, the neighborhood, the school, and the community. One crucial decision that often takes place early in treatment is which parts of the social environment to include directly in the treatment. Various groups of individuals can be included for assessment only or may be more involved in the ongoing treatment.

3. *Negotiating the goals of treatment:* The family or couple usually comes to treatment with their own goals in mind. Unlike individual therapy, however, in which one individual comes with his or her own goals, the family comes with a few individuals having specific goals, often for other people (not themselves) to change, and some individuals not wanting to be there at all.

■ DISTRIBUTION OF TIME

If one is engaged in short-term crisis intervention, 30 minutes may be all the time that is available for evaluation. Joining must be done quickly, evaluation is done only for the presenting problem, and further evaluation occurs during the intervention. In a training or practice setting, with no fixed time limit for treatment, one may be able to allot more time for thorough evaluation, such as a quick genogram. Some clinicians take the time at an initial phone contact to gather detailed biographical and historical information. This may save time initially but is not a substitute for a thorough and complete interview with the entire family.

■ BUILDING A TREATMENT ALLIANCE

Styles and techniques of gathering history are very much related to the crucial task of building a treatment alliance with the family.

These techniques vary as to which phase of the treatment is operative. This ground was covered earlier in this book, but some of it will be repeated here in the context of course of treatment.

We recommend that most therapists obtain a fairly extensive history, perhaps mainly in the opening sessions. Some family therapy models, such as those that are solution focused, prefer a less extensive history diagnosis and more emphasis on the here and now, working more with what happens in the session and gathering longitudinal data only as needed during the course of the meetings.

The therapist may decide to hear from each family member in turn on certain important issues or may allow the verbal interaction to take its own course. It is important to allow for at least a few minutes of unguided conversation among family members in order to observe their patterns of interaction. However, it is demoralizing to the family to allow a fight to continue for too long, once the pattern of the fight has been seen. A decision may be made to call on one parent first, then the other, and then the children in descending chronological order. In other instances it may appear more advantageous to call on the more easily intimidated, weaker, or passive parent (or spouse) first, or to allow the family to decide who speaks first. The therapist may decide to use first names for all family members to help put everyone on an equal footing, or he or she may prefer to be more formal in addressing the parents in order to strengthen relatively weak generational boundaries and parental functioning. Some therapists may encourage the family members to talk with one another, whereas others may focus family members' conversation largely through the therapist, at least during the first sessions or at times of stress or chaos.

The assumption is made that the family's behavior in sessions and at home is similar. This is not always true, however, since the family's behavior is usually modified in some ways in sessions by the presence of the therapist. In the beginning, the therapist is something of an outsider, whose main function may be to allow everyone, including the weakest members of the family, to be heard. Some family members are often on the attack, whereas others are defensive during the initial period. An identified patient who is an adolescent often demands changes at home, because individuals in this age group are frequently the ones most interested in change. An angry, frustrated spouse may demand that the marital partner change. Some therapists may point out that they will not be decision makers for the family but will help the family members clarify their problems and help them with their decision-making processes. Such therapists may act as referees or traffic cops when necessary, making sure that one person speaks at a time, that no one person is overwhelmed by attacks during the sessions, and that nonconstructive family patterns are not allowed to continue unchallenged during the therapy sessions. They create an atmosphere that encourages the verbal expression of feelings toward constructive ends.

Therapists indicate that in an unhappy family, everyone hurts and therefore everyone wants to get something positive out of the sessions. A therapist conveys the feeling that all the family members are doing the best they can and that one needs to understand the motives of oneself and of others. Nevertheless, the family therapist explains that well-intentioned attitudes and actions are nevertheless sometimes less than totally positive in their outcomes.

Families vary considerably in their readiness to move from a discussion of the current crisis situation to an exploration of their patterns and histories. Therapists will follow the family's lead in these respects; for instance, a couple may refuse to discuss an issue that exists between them, focusing only on the children. In other cases, a therapist may be willing to start the sessions even though the father is absent and may sense that the family members need some time to talk about the badness of one of the offspring.

It is important for the therapist to get an idea of the family's mode of operation in order to convey a sense of respect for and understanding of the family's initial point of view. At the same time, the therapist should guard against being so passive and accepting that nothing new will be added to the equation. The family's experience in the therapy hour should not be merely a repetition of the nongratifying interactional patterns for which they originally sought help. It may be helpful to tell the family that individual problems are often related to family problems and that they all need to find out more about the family as a whole to enable each member, and the family as an entity, to benefit from the treatment.

When speaking of choice points, it may be desirable to move on to a longitudinal, chronological narrative of the family's history (perhaps through three generations) or, alternatively, to begin with a cross-sectional inventory of how the family currently functions. Which of these areas will be discussed first depends on the therapist's predilections, the family's distress, and the nature of the difficulty. The major longitudinal data to be gathered will refer to the parents' period of courtship, engagement, marriage, honeymoon, early years of marriage before the arrival of children, and the changes in the family as a result of the first child, each subsequent child, and so on through the family cycle.

One may start with the courtship period (which is, in part, predictive of marital patterns), move on to the marriage, and then work backward, having each partner review his or her original family. One can discuss the life history before the marriage for each partner, including any previous marriages. In going back to the parents' families of origin, one gets a picture of the functioning of those previous families that serves as a foundation for understanding the present family and its problems. Careful attention must be given not only to recollections of the past and expressions regarding attitudes and values, but also to overt behavior. A complete sexual history should carefully delineate difficulties in sexual adjustment. It is our experience that this is something still done all too rarely in the field of family therapy, as though sexual problems were regarded as only secondary to other interpersonal difficulties. However, the timing of obtaining the sexual history is critical, even with presenting sexual problems. Two rules of thumb are that obtaining the history of sexual problems 1) should usually wait until other history is known and 2) is best not begun in the last half hour of the session. Sexual history taking should not be done with children present.

■ SPECIAL ISSUES IN EVALUATION

Although we have discussed evaluation earlier in this text and re-visit it in the next section on couples treatment, we emphasize a few points here for the purpose of elucidating some special issues that affect the course of therapy. Each of the following topics is discussed in greater detail in subsequent chapters; we mention them here only in the context of the course of treatment.

Sexuality

Primary difficulties in sexual adjustment often sour the rest of the marital relationship. Sometimes sexual difficulties are the major area of difficulty for the married couple and perhaps the one most difficult for them to deal with. Some couples appear to need and benefit from specific therapy directed toward improving their sexual adjustment. To the extent that this can be done satisfactorily, other areas of marital and family interaction may then markedly improve. The sexual adjustment of the marital pair should be evaluated as carefully as other areas of marital and family interaction. It is not safe to assume that any sexual problems are secondary and will always resolve themselves more or less spontaneously when other areas of family difficulty have been overcome. Needless to say, parents' sexuality is not usually discussed in the presence of the children. With teenagers, the particulars of their sexual experience are also discussed in private, but families need to discuss the guidelines for adolescent sexual behavior within the family. It is the task of the family therapist to 1) set the guidelines for discussion and 2) help the family clearly state their beliefs on sexual activity, sexual safety, and respect and love for the partner.

Money

Another area often overlooked or slighted in the evaluation phase is that of the family's dealings with money. We have found this to be an important issue in marital and family friction. As with sexuality, the issue of money is not always merely secondary to other marital problems. Some marital couples have never been able to work out a satisfactory way of managing money as a marital pair. Any other marital problem may be reflected in fights about money, just as problems may be reflected in sexual maladjustment.

Gender

All couples operate within a larger social system in which men are generally privileged, but couples' individual ways of dealing with differences in power and gender-based communication vary greatly. The interviewer needs to gain an understanding early on of whether men or women are devalued in a particular family and what kinds of power are available to each partner.

Ethnicity

Where the interviewer may see subtle ethnic differences, the participants may see major fault lines. For example, Irish Catholics and Italian Catholics have some very different traditions about home and family. Couples who have crossed ethnic, racial, or class lines in their marriage may have extra stresses, either because of such issues between themselves or because of disapproval within their families of origin.

Individual Diagnoses

The interviewer must be alert to the possibility of major mental illness, addiction, or dysthymia in one or more family members. Couples in which both partners have a mood disorder are not uncommon. The interviewer must decide in what context to conduct an individual diagnostic workup.

Phase of the Family Life Cycle

The amount and type of data to be assembled will be strongly influenced by the current phase of the family life cycle. It is appropriate to concentrate on material that is relevant to issues pertaining to that particular phase of family life. The relative emphasis, as well as some of the specific content of the history to be gathered, would be quite different if one were dealing with a couple in the first year of marriage or a family whose last offspring is preparing to leave home.

Should the therapist allow the family to present the history, or should he or she structure the history with an outline? Most therapists seem to combine both approaches. It is often helpful to let the family members talk until they have told their story in their own way. On the other hand, the therapist has expertise in helping families with problems and can help them in structuring a history. What is not mentioned or does not emerge because of the structuring, we believe, will emerge with time, but what is missed by not asking (for example, not taking a sexual history) may never be revealed.

■ EVALUATION VERSUS TREATMENT

For clarity of presentation we have separated family evaluation and family treatment. In practice, this rarely happens and is not particularly desirable. A process of continual evaluation and hypothesis testing takes place throughout the course of therapy, and the therapist constantly checks his or her perceptions. At the same time, every session should have some beneficial outcome. The more skillful and experienced the therapist and the less rigid the approach, the more total the blend of evaluative and therapeutic aspects and the more extensive the use of improvised variations, condensations, and extensions on some of the themes.

> Mr. and Mrs. M, a young couple in their early twenties, came for treatment because their marriage was in trouble. An evaluation was done (using the format described in Chapter 7). At the beginning of the session the following week, the therapist asked the couple what had happened since the evaluation. Mr. M said he realized that they were not communicating, but they had made a point of increasing communication during the week. Mrs. M said that she thought the session had not done anything, but she had recognized for the first time that there was a communication problem.

■ EARLY PHASE

During the early phase of treatment, the therapist comes to a better understanding of the life of the family, making contact and promoting empathy and communication. Some major nonproductive patterns are spotlighted, and scapegoating is neutralized. A process is begun in which the focus is moved away from the identified patient and attention is directed to the entire family system. (See Table 8–1 for the objectives of treatment in the early phase.)

TABLE 8–1. **Objectives of the early phase**

1. Detail the primary problems and nonproductive family patterns.
2. Clarify the goals for treatment.
3. Solidify the therapeutic contract.
4. Strengthen the therapeutic relationship.
5. Shift the focus from the identified patient to the entire family system.
6. Decrease guilt and blame.
7. Increase the ability of family members to empathize with one another.
8. Assess the family's strengths.
9. Assess the family's preferred style of thinking and working.
10. Define who is in the family.
11. Obtain a clear idea of what ethnic and cultural issues are part of the family's functioning.
12. Determine the life cycle phase for each individual and for the family.

■ MIDDLE PHASE

The middle stage is often considered to be the one in which the major work of change takes place. What the therapist does during the middle stage varies depending on the goals that have been singled out as being of primary importance. Common examples of persistent, nongratifying interpersonal patterns and attitudes, preferably drawn from recent or here-and-now interactions, are repeatedly discussed. Old nonfunctional coalitions, rules, myths, and role models are challenged, and the possibility of alternative modes is presented. New habits of thinking, feeling, and interacting take time to develop, and much repetition is often required. At the same time, resistance to change comes to the fore and must be dealt with accordingly.

The initial focus may be on the identified patient, but the focus then moves to the family. Often the identified patient may improve before the family does.

A crisis often develops when problems that have been hidden away or have been too painful to face are brought to the conscious awareness of the family members.

> In the N family, the identified patient was Mr. N, who had chronic anxiety and depression. Mrs. N was a loyal but suffering housewife. There were two young children. Mrs. N had been doing most of the child rearing. The couple socialized very little. When the family was brought together, Mr. N talked about his wife's chronic hostility toward him. She responded by saying, "Look what I put up with." As communication finally opened up over a period of weeks, the anger escalated until the couple was talking about divorce. This crisis was used to change the patterns of family participation on the part of both parents. Mr. N, after starting medications, began to share some of the family tasks, such as getting the children to school on time and helping them to do their homework. Mrs. N had more time for herself. She returned to work as a biochemist. Feeling better about herself and about her husband's ability to be part of the family, she suggested to her husband that they go out to movies and concerts.

In early stages of therapy, the situation may appear to worsen, rather than improve. The therapist must monitor the situation carefully and frame the situation as potentially positive. In the middle stages, symptomatology may accelerate, new symptoms may arise, and families may talk about quitting treatment. This upheaval is usually related to the family's barely perceived awareness that, for the situation to get better, some member will have to change. Rather than change, a family member may accentuate or exaggerate symptoms. Family therapy changes have to be made sequentially. For example, a family cannot let go of an offspring until the marital couple has found increased satisfaction in their own lives and in their relationship.

At the start of therapy, it is crucial for the therapist to meet the family where they are coming from and gradually draw them toward the therapeutic scenario. Figure 8–1 presents a schematic diagram to illustrate this process, which occurs gradually.

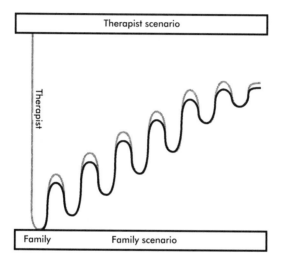

FIGURE 8–1. **Schematic of the joining of therapist and family scenarios.**
Source. Concept courtesy of Marion Forgatch, Oregon Social Learning Center, 1997.

On the bottom line of Figure 8–1, it can be seen that the family has their own scenario and, left to their own devices, they follow patterns that are scripted, repetitive, and unchanging. Similarly, at the top of the diagram, the therapist has his or her scenario of what he or she thinks the problem is. The same can hold true for the therapist as for the family—that is, without interaction with the family, that scenario does not vary. The essence of the therapy is to bring together the two scenarios, beginning at the top left of the diagram, as the therapist and the family interact. Presumably, the family's behavior changes as they interact, using the therapist's strategies. The diagram also points out that therapy is never a smooth line. As it continues, there are always spurts, retreats, and frequent oscillations, but therapy should be moving forward to achieve the goals that were set up earlier.

■ TERMINATION PHASE

In the closing phase, the therapist reviews with the family which goals have and have not been achieved. It is often useful to review the entire course of therapy, including the original problems and goals. A useful technique is to ask each family member to state what he or she would have to do to make the situation the same as it was at the onset of treatment. For example, the father would have to yell at the mother, who would have to yell at the daughter, who would have to stop going to school. In essence, the family reconstructs the sequences leading to the pathology. Videotape playback may be helpful at this time so that the family can see what it looked like at the start of treatment compared with its present stage. It is important to acknowledge that some behavior cannot be altered and that life will continue to change—that is, to have unexpected and periodic problems. The family should be provided with the skills for solving future conflicts and challenges.

What are the criteria for suggesting termination of therapy? If the original goals have been achieved, the therapist may consider stopping. When the treatment has been successful, new coping patterns and an enhanced empathy by family members for one another will have been established. There will be recognition that the family itself seems capable of dealing satisfactorily with new situations as they arise. There may be little to talk about during the sessions and little sense of urgency. Nonproductive quarreling and conflict will have been reduced; the family members will be freer to disagree openly and will have methods of living with and working out their differences and separateness. The family will seem less inflexible in its rules and organization and appear more able to grow and develop. Individual family members will be symptomatically improved, and positive channels of interaction will be available between all family members. There will be improved agreement about family roles and functions.

Even if the goals have not been achieved but have been worked out to the best capabilities of therapist and family, therapy can stop. If the therapist feels stuck but believes more change is possible, it is helpful to obtain a consultation before ending therapy.

Families often cannot or do not recognize changes that have occurred during therapy. A therapist should carefully check for any change and amplify it, giving positive reinforcement. If a family can produce a small change, this may be an indication that bigger changes are possible. With some families, no change may occur until the therapy is completed.

Often after successful therapy, when termination issues have been resolved, the family has a resurgence of symptoms. This usually indicates anxiety over ending rather than a new problem. The family is encouraged to have the symptoms to determine whether there are any that they want to keep. If they say no, they are encouraged to watch to see how symptoms occur and review what happens on the days when symptoms do not occur. They are encouraged to see this as a review or a final examination.

During this end phase, there may be an exacerbation of presenting symptoms. A son may begin hallucinating again coincident with the father's reduction in communication with the mother (after losing his job), or the son may stop taking his medications and begin hallucinating, and the couple may begin arguing about it. These eruptions are usually short lived and may represent a temporary response to the anxiety of terminating treatment rather than being a sign of treatment failure. The eruptions are thus part of the separation process, which is always a key issue to be worked on in termination and which in some theoretical orientations may represent the major theme of the entire therapy.

9

PROMOTING CHANGE IN FAMILY TREATMENT: ISSUES OF ALLIANCE AND RESISTANCE

In this chapter we discuss two issues that may not seem related—the therapeutic alliance and resistance. By *therapeutic alliance,* we mean the collaborative relationship between the family therapist and the family that is aimed at promoting change. By resistance, we mean the processes in the patient or the family that impede change. Both are central to the process of therapy, and without the first, the alliance, it is almost impossible to deal with the second, resistance.

■ THE THERAPEUTIC ALLIANCE

The family unit is often portrayed as sanctified. Certainly, popular politics touts it thus, celebrating the importance of family values as a means to alleviate a wide variety of societal ills. The therapist is an outsider, initially unaware of the family's complex (and often dysfunctional) rules. To alter the system, one must first be accepted by the system.

The success of any therapeutic endeavor depends on the participants establishing and maintaining an open, trusting, and collaborative relationship or alliance. In couple and family therapy, the therapeutic alliance offers the opportunity for corrective experience and is a necessary condition for therapeutic change. A growing body of empirical evidence demonstrates that the therapeutic alliance is the best predictor of psychotherapy outcome in individual therapy, and a similar line of clinical research in relation to couple and family treatment has begun to emerge. The functions of a therapeutic alliance include instilling hope in the family and creating an environment that is safe enough for the family to engage in new behaviors that take them past their comfort zone. The family must believe that the therapist not only has the skills to help them through the problem but also respects and appreciates them as people. Issues for the family therapist in establishing an alliance include the following:

- One must form an alliance with several people at once, who often have quite different feelings and agendas.
- One must keep in mind the need to adopt a conceptual framework to account for interactions within triangles, or systems of three (or more) persons.
- The system will operate in powerful ways to induct the therapist into it.
- The fact that multiple participants are present means that people with different motivations, goals, and beliefs about how to change must all be attended to. If the participant has come involuntarily, as with many adolescents and most court-ordered patients, the situation is even more complicated.

Sessions with any family tend to be more complex and more openly conflicted than do most individual sessions. The therapist must work to develop a connection with each person, with the various subsystems, and with the family as a whole. In this process, the therapist must be constantly aware of the presence of triangles among family members and among himself or herself and family members: no dyadic relationship in therapy can exist outside a series of interlocking triangles. This means that, for example, if the therapist develops a strong relationship with one spouse, the other may feel left out or angry. Any move the therapist makes may be seen from a variety of different angles.

The therapist who joins the system experiences the pull of the system—that is, the request to operate within the system's rules and beliefs—to help the family change the problem without changing the system. This process is subtle and very strong. If the therapist, for example, buys into the family's definition of the problem as "we have a bad child," he or she may not pay attention to the marital problem or the problems of the child who is labeled good. The therapist must see the constraints on behavior (this cannot be talked about, this cannot be changed) as information to use in understanding the system and must remain separate enough not to be bound by these constraints.

Alliance formation for the therapist is complicated by multiple countertransferential reactions. The therapist may be drawn to or may prefer some members of the family. Family dynamics may replicate the therapist's family in some way, producing wishes to save or to punish certain family members. In addition, the therapist can see how badly one person is treating another, as one does not in individual therapy. When watching a parent verbally abuse a child in session, it is difficult to find a way to ally with the parent as well as the child; yet unless the therapist can connect with all family members in some way, the family will extrude him or her.

Different family theorists use different forms of connection and joining, which are related to their overall model. Satir and Baldwin (1983), for example, modeled warmth, support, and respect for give-and-take and emphasized that therapist and patients were equals in learning. In his model, Bowen (1978) took the position that the therapist is coach or researcher and kept more distant to avoid being affected by the family's emotional process. The model of Haley and Hoffman (1967) and many solution-focused models use the therapist's position as expert. These models differ in the use of the therapist's power and the level of appropriate closeness. At one end are therapists who see themselves as defining the problem and having the job of fixing it, whereas at the other end are coconstructors of a new reality, who are quite humble about their suggestions. The position that a particular therapist chooses will relate to his or her model of therapy, specific personality, and situation. Different therapists, by virtue of their positions with certain patients, will be able to take some positions more easily than others. For example, a 50-year-old male M.D. will be more able to take an expert or "uncle" position than will a 25-year-old female social worker, who might work more effectively from a position of one down or from a conversational model or an equals-in-learning model.

■ MODELS FOR DEALING WITH FAMILIES WHO HAVE TROUBLE FORMING AN ALLIANCE

In the family therapy field there are currently at least four different models for dealing with families who present difficulties in forming a therapeutic alliance: 1) the medical model, 2) the coaching model, 3) the conflict model, and 4) the strategic systems model. These models are described in the following paragraphs.

The Medical Model

In the medical model, it is assumed that the index patient has an illness, such as schizophrenia or major affective disorder, and that the family is not the only, or necessarily the principal, factor in the etiology of the illness. With this assumption, the major strategy in reducing family resistance to treatment is psychoeducation for the family, in which they are taught about the symptoms, etiology, and course of the illness. In this model, it is emphasized that the family did not cause the illness, thus reducing family guilt and resistance to meeting with the therapist. The family therapist takes on the role of a teacher who instructs the family about the illness and what the family can do to ensure optimal coping.

The Coaching Model

Therapists who work in both individual and family formats using behavioral techniques tended until recently to ignore the concept of resistance in their writings. Instead, they emphasized that individuals in families must learn certain basic social, communication, and negotiating skills for harmonious interactions and that individuals lacked these skills because of gaps in prior learning. In this model, it was assumed that the therapist was a coach and rational collaborator who elicited the cooperation of the patient and family in learning missing skills. More recently, behavioral therapists have become interested in the issues of what prevents the learning of these skills. They have developed cognitive-behavioral models in which the role of the cognitive meaning of behaviors is considered, so that resistance is also examined as a series of cognitive distortions and beliefs that impede learning ("If I'm nice to her and give in, I won't be a real man"; "He is really a bad person, so why should I give him anything?").

In a coaching model, it is assumed that the therapist helps the couple to locate problem areas and to address them in a rational and focused way. Resistance to learning skills, such as failure to do homework or diverting attention in the session from practice, may be met first with rational argument ("You need these skills to function well"), encouragement, and positive reinforcement. However, therapists also work with the couple or family to uncover distortions and replace dysfunctional cognitions with more functional ones.

The Conflict Model

In a continuation of the psychodynamic tradition, the conflict model assumes that particular individuals in the marital or family system may resist intervention and change on the basis of their own internal conflicts and defense mechanisms. In this model, the family therapist, like the individual dynamic therapist, uses techniques of confrontation and interpretation of the here-and-now interaction, especially negative interactions that might destroy the therapeutic relationship and the very survival of the therapy itself.

The Strategic Systems Model

A unique contribution of the family field is its theoretical position regarding the strength of a pattern of family interactions that shape and mold the behavior and psychopathology of an individual member of that group. In this orientation, it is assumed that family systems in homeostasis, even when the homeostasis involves severe problems, will resist change. When faced with resistance of a whole system, the therapist may use strategic interventions to change not individual behaviors but a pattern of systems behaviors.

■ DIFFICULTIES IN CREATING CHANGE: DISCONNECTION AND RESISTANCE

Resistance in family therapy is usually defined as forces within the patient or family that impede apparently wished-for change. Although resistance is usually seen as negative, it is also clear that personal and family stability depend on certain consistencies of thought and behavior, so psychological mechanisms and family rules are not designed for instant change. In general, families are likely to have an idea of what changes they want to make and are confused about why they cannot do these things. The task of the therapist and family then becomes to understand the specific ideas and fears that stand in the way of change. Some families are not open to change at any level at a particular point in time. However, lack of change in therapy is often attributed to family mechanisms when the real problem is a disconnect between therapist and patients, meaning that the therapist is not correctly assessing the system or has lost the family's trust. In summary, problems in creating change during therapy can come from the family, from disconnects in the family-therapist system, or primarily from the therapist (inexperience, mistakes in judgment, etc.).

Problems in Change: Within the System

Families fear change for many reasons. Most problem behaviors were originally adaptive mechanisms that are now failing but that are frightening to let go of unless there is something to put in their place. For example, if an overly close relationship between a daughter and a mother made up for the mother's poor marital relationship with her husband, the mother will need to believe that she can change the relationship with her husband, or can feel better herself, before she can wholeheartedly let go of her daughter. If a father believes that his son will be a sissy unless the father yells at him and bullies him, the father will have to change that belief before he can change his behavior.

Sometimes the family has a toxic secret that they are afraid to reveal. For example, no one may be willing to speak about a father's sexual abuse of his daughter because they are afraid that he will retaliate with violence, so they are unable to mobilize themselves to change any of the resulting problems.

Certain conditions in individuals make change far more complex. For example, alcoholism and drug addiction sometimes respond to family interventions, but if they do not, only limited change is possible. Similarly, with severe mental illness in a parent, appropriate psychiatric medical management must accompany family therapy or the situation will be very difficult to change.

Problems in Change: Therapist Induced

Therapists face many challenges as they begin to deal with a family, including their own powerful countertransference feelings. Therapists who become angry at or too connected to some members of the family will be unable to form an alliance with the whole system, which is necessary for change. Therapists may blame the family for the symptoms of one member, as did many early practitioners dealing with schizophrenia, making their hostility so apparent that the family members were unable to take anything useful from them.

In addition, therapist mistakes will make it appear that the family is resisting. For example, failing to diagnose attention-deficit/hyperactivity disorder in a child, the therapist may insist that the problem is an overprotective mother and spend time working to get her less involved, when the child actually needs both medication and more structure. If a couple presents with wife abuse and the therapist concentrates on communication and does not directly interdict the husband's violence, it is unlikely that much will change.

In addition, even if the therapist correctly understands the family system, he or she will be unable to help the family to move forward if he or she is unable to control the session, fails to give tasks that are small enough and clear enough for learning to occur, is not clear about goals and directions, or does not explain his or her theory to the family.

Problems in Change: Stemming From the Relationship Between Therapist and System

Mismatch Between Therapist and Family

Although most therapists learn to work with a variety of patients over time, some therapist-patient systems are too difficult to manage, especially with beginning therapists. For example, a very young female therapist who was newly married was assigned to work with a midlife couple in sex therapy. The wife, who was depressed, angry, and feeling unlovable because of years of sexual disinterest on the part of her husband, could not stand being treated by a woman she saw as a rival and who in addition did not have the life experience to understand midlife issues. The couple did well when transferred to an older therapist who could connect more directly with the couple's life experience and circumstances. Sometimes the therapist's style of functioning is too far from the needs of the patient system—too aggressive, passive, or distant.

Disagreement as to Goals of Treatment

Problems can also occur when the therapist believes one goal is central and the family wishes another. For example, the therapist may see couple issues as critical, whereas the family wishes to talk only about the child. If the therapist moves too fast or does not wait to see whether the family has accepted the new goal, treatment will stall.

Failure to Include Those Outside the Nuclear Family

The system may include others besides the nuclear family, and the therapist may not take this into account. Common systems to be considered include family elders, such as grandparents or other relatives, who may have very definite ideas about what should be done, as well as the school system, the legal system, and, if a family member is also physically ill, the medical system. Multiproblem families are often involved with several caregivers who may have very different ideas about the problem and its solution. Such situations may involve child welfare, the school, a social worker, legal services, or other therapists seeing family members. If the therapist is working in an agency, another set of systems is involved. For example, the family may be very suspicious of therapists in social welfare or probation, seeing them as agents of social control rather than support. A therapist's supervisor or agency rules may be in conflict with the treatment the family or the therapist wishes.

Problems in Change: By Phase of Treatment at Evaluation and Early in Treatment

The first task of the therapist is to set the structure within which the family intervention can occur, and during this process of negotiating the structure with the family, many resistances can surface. In contrast to individual therapy, family or marital therapy necessitates the attendance of a number of people, most of whom do not have overt symptoms. The therapist must first decide whether to insist on seeing the whole family.

At times it is best to begin work with whoever comes to treatment first and support them in getting the rest of the family to come. In general it is best to insist on seeing the whole family as close to the beginning of therapy as possible.

Strategies for getting members of the family involved include the following: reassuring the missing member of his or her importance, pointing out that changes depend on his or her presence, noting that his or her absence can sabotage therapy, providing flexibility in scheduling, and spacing appointments (Anderson and Stewart 1983; Napier and Whitaker 1978). A number of principles ensure attendance in starting family intervention with drug addicts and their families (they are probably appropriate for other symptom groups as well):

- The therapist, not the family, should decide which family members will be included in the treatment.
- Whenever possible, family members should be encouraged to attend the evaluation interview.
- The index patient (or the *identified patient*) alone should not be given the task of bringing in the other members of the family.
- The therapist should obtain permission from the index patient and should personally contact the family (fathers in particular should be contacted personally).
- The therapist should contact the family with a rationale for family intervention that is nonpejorative and nonjudgmental and in no way blames the family for the symptoms and problems of the index patient.

Often the critical issue is in supporting the overtly symptomatic patient to ask for help from the family.

> In the O family, Mr. O was the identified patient, with a long history of unipolar depression. Once his depressive episodes had been regulated with medication, he told the therapist that his wife was unhappy with their relationship. The therapist suggested marital therapy. Mr. O stated that this was "his cross to bear," because she would not come in for therapy. The therapist suggested that he try again to talk to her about this. Mrs. O surprisingly appeared for the next session and stated that she was unhappy with the relationship but had never been asked to come in for therapy. Mr. O stated that he had asked her but admitted he might have "mumbled the invitation."

Families in which a member exhibits current self-destructive behaviors (e.g., suicidal threats, gestures, and attempts; anorexia and/or bulimia; drug abuse; physical violence) present special issues in the initial structuring of the therapy. The therapist must often spell out in great detail what he or she will and will not do when these behaviors occur. The therapist can also help the family members to plan how they will behave. If this is not done, the first resistance will come in the form of destructive behaviors that derail the possibility of change.

As we have said earlier, another area of potential resistance and deadlock in the early phase is disagreement about the goals of treatment. We began the discussion of this issue in Chapter 8 in our discussion of the process of bringing together both the family's and the therapists' views (i.e., scenario) of the problem. The family members themselves may disagree about the problem and the goals of treatment. For example, the family of an index adolescent patient may see the adolescent as the only problem, whereas the adolescent sees no problem in himself or herself and sees the parents as authoritarian, narrow, and hostile. In marital therapy, covert disagreement about the problem, and especially about the goals of intervention, may occur when one spouse wants to improve the marriage while the other secretly wants out, is intending to leave the spouse, and wants the therapist to assist in the breakup.

Strategies to overcome family differences about the problem include searching for a new definition of the problem with which all family members agree, labeling the disagreement as part of the problem, and asking the family to give up idiosyncratic notions about their version of truth and reality. Encouraging family members to say what has remained unsaid can approach covert goals. Disagreement about the goals of intervention can also occur between the therapist and the family. This seems most prominent when the therapist sees the problems of the index patient as related to the interactions of the family, while the family sees no contribution of their own and wants the index patient changed or cured. The therapist can approach this problem by initially accepting the family's view of the problem, or at least not challenging it, or by broadening the family's definition to include other aspects of interaction.

When a family member has been hospitalized for the first time with the initial emergence of psychotic symptomatology diagnosed as either schizophrenia or mood disorder, a common resistance of the family is to deny either the presence of this illness or its severity. If such denial persists, the family is in danger of avoiding follow-up care for the patient and family and of furthering expectations for the index patient that are unrealistic and thus stressful for the vulnerable individual.

A particularly troublesome resistance for the beginning family therapist, especially if he or she is a psychiatric resident, psychology intern, or social work student, is the family's attack on the therapist's competence or personal characteristics (e.g., age, sex, race, socioeconomic level, etc.). These resistances can come in subtle barrages ("You're so good for a youngster, but you probably don't know much about older people") and not-so-subtle barrages ("This is probably your first case, and we are not making any progress. Have you talked to your supervisor about this?"). Contact with an experienced and level-headed supervisor is most helpful in these situations. If the therapist is able to see these remarks in the context of resistance, he or she can explore the meaning of the questions about competence by empathizing with the family's concern. With equilibrium and, at times, humor, the therapist can admit differences and limitations (youth, relative inexperience), appeal to the family for their assistance and help, and ask for a period in which to give the therapy a chance to succeed.

However, if it is clear that the family cannot tolerate the situation, transfer to a therapist whom they have requested (older, younger, different race or gender) is indicated. Either the family was correct in its assessment that they needed something different, or once they have proved they have some control in a situation, it may be safe for them to begin work.

Problems in Change: By Phase of Treatment in Ongoing Treatment

It is extremely common for a therapy to move rapidly in the early weeks and then stall. This is the point at which old habits reassert themselves, the natural homeostasis of the family takes over, and small failures begin to seem insurmountable. The process of working through change is difficult. The therapist needs to review the treatment and decide whether to change direction or to simply support the idea that change is sometimes difficult and to continue in the same direction.

Anderson and Stewart (1983) have listed a number of interests that threaten treatment: a family member who is consistently too talkative and dominant; a family member who refuses to speak; chaotic and disruptive children; use of defenses such as intellectualization, rationalization, and denial; constant focus by one or more members on placing blame on others; or unwillingness to perform assigned tasks or homework necessary for change. The therapist can limit overly talkative members or can encourage other family members to do so. Parents of chaotic children can be educated by words and the model of the therapist to set controls in the sessions. Most important is the therapist's understanding of why the behavior is occurring. If the behavior serves a purpose, it will be less amenable to requests to discontinue it unless the underlying meaning is addressed. However, if the therapist can create a different experience in the session, such as getting a quiet husband to talk while his wife listens, the family may be able to repeat the experience at home without needing to have specific insight into why things have changed.

When couples argue as a regular pattern, usually they are not trying to understand what the other is saying. It is more likely that they are feeling defensive and out of control, so they listen for weaknesses in logic to leap on or selectively mishear what the partner says. Such couples misread each other's intent, feel defensive, and believe that if they don't attack first, they will be injured. Behind this is a deep sense of hurt. The truth is more likely to be found in the complex middle than in the simplified extremes. Therefore, the therapist must discuss the process of the argument and its underlying meanings.

If tasks are not being done, the therapist can challenge the couple or redesign the task. Refusal to do homework should always be discussed, because in the discussion are the cues about what is really going on.

There are a number of techniques for handling defenses, not unlike those one might use in individual or group therapy. To counteract intellectualization and rationalization, the therapist can go with the theme by emphasizing the intellectual aspects of the therapy and/or giving intellectual explanations. Relabeling of feelings as facts may help. A denying family can be slowed down so as to emphasize aspects before they are glossed over. Nonverbal and experiential techniques can also be used to get to denied material. Finally, as a last resort, the therapist can focus on and support a no-change position as a way to eventually get change.

Resistance by Phase: At the Ending Stages of Therapy

As stated in Chapter 8, often, after successful therapy, as termination begins, the family has a resurgence of symptoms resulting from anxiety over termination. The family can use this time to review their progress and to further understand their issues. They may be encouraged to have the symptoms to see if there are any that they would like to keep. They may use the situation to track the symptoms to understand how they occur and when they are avoided, so as to lock in new behaviors. However, the therapist should be alert to the idea that the family is asking for more support and should plan appropriate follow-up care.

Family Secrets

Individuals in the family often have secrets that in most cases are known but not acknowledged by other family members. These secrets may involve overt behaviors, such as marital infidelity, that one marital partner feels he or she has been able to conceal from the other; or they may involve thoughts, feelings, and attitudes that family members believe others are not aware of. For example, parents may not realize (or may deny) that children pick up the general emotional tone existing between mother and father. They may act as though marital discord is hidden from their children and may want to keep that discord secret. The family can also keep secrets hidden from the therapist.

> The P family consisted of a hospitalized adolescent, the parents, and two older siblings. For 10 weeks, the family therapy seemed to be bogged down. The family stopped treatment. Two months later, the family therapist discovered a secret that the entire family already knew—that is, the identified patient was having sexual

relations with a ward nurse. The patient had told his siblings, who told the parents, who then signed the patient out of the hospital. The secret served the purpose of denigrating the hospital staff (including the family therapist) and effectively halting the family therapy.

Helping the family bring these pseudosecrets into the open usually results in a clearing of the air and eventually leads to a sense of relief and greater mutual understanding. Interestingly, it is commonly the children who talk openly in family sessions about what was thought by others to be a secret. The therapist should, however, be prepared to deal with acute shock waves at the time the secret first emerges. When an individual in a family requests an individual session for the purpose of revealing a secret, the therapist may listen and try to explore the consequences of discussing the issue within the family setting. If, for example, one of the spouses has an incurable illness and the other spouse does not know about it, the reasons for the secrecy would be examined and the spouse would be encouraged to share the information with the whole family. If the secret does not seem critical to the relationship, the therapist might take a more neutral stance. (For a good discussion of secrets and the distinction between secrets and power, see Imber-Black [1993].) The therapist must guard against being trapped into becoming a repository of secrets and has the right to tell the patient the therapy will end unless the secret is told.

At times a family member may insist on total honesty, either because of emotional insensitivity or as an active way of hurting another family member. For example, a parent might report to a child every negative feeling that crosses his or her mind in the guise of honesty.

It is not recommended that therapists themselves reveal a family secret unless a no-confidentiality clause has been agreed to in advance.

A therapist who finds a family to be resistant can take several steps, as shown in Table 9–1.

In the same vein, Alves (1992) has suggested that therapists often refer to their patient families as being "stuck" when movement

---

TABLE 9–1.   **Techniques for dealing with resistance in stalled therapy**

Announce to the family that the therapist feels stuck and ask if the family does.   Sometimes the family is actually doing fine and only the therapist is anxious. If everyone feels stuck, then everyone can work on the problem together.

Retake a history.   The most common reason for problems in therapy is that the therapist does not have all the facts and so has not properly formulated the problem or the solution. Some information is not shared with therapists until late in therapy, when the patients are more trusting. Sometimes if a family came in crisis, the original history was too sketchy. The best way to regroup is to start over, preferably with a more complete genogram related to the problem.

Go up or down a system level.   Often the problem, or the solution, is involving more people. If one is seeing a couple, one can go up a level by involving more people—their children or their parents. One can go down a level by doing some individual work.

Do the opposite of what you have been doing.   With therapy, as with life, sometimes the solution becomes the problem. If pushing hard does not work, prescribe the symptom.[a] If you have been gentle and nonconfrontational, try pushing harder.

Obtain a consultation.   A consultation serves notice to everyone that there is a problem and opens the system up for new ways of thinking. Consultants can often see a problem or blind spot because they are less connected to the family system and can visualize the therapist-family system as a whole.

---

[a]Prescribe the symptom: the therapist asks the family member to intensify or increase the frequency of a symptom. The aim is to make the symptom alien or foreign so as to eventually stop the behavior.

---

in the therapy process breaks down. Often when this occurs, it is the therapist who has gotten off track and contributed to, if not directly reinforced, the lack of progress. Therapists have a major responsibility to get the therapy process back on track. A return to a few basic, fundamental principles often dislodges even the most stubborn roadblocks to progress. Following are a few trusty standbys on which we rely.

- *Assume nothing:* As we have said, it goes without saying that a thorough assessment of a family's presenting problems and overall functioning is key to the therapy process. However, problems in therapy presented in supervision can often be traced back to a hurried, haphazard assessment. Therapists either do not ask all the questions or jump to conclusions based on limited information. Assumptions made by therapists about family treatment goals typically create blocks to progress if the family has not agreed to such goals. A quick check of this area often reveals that what the therapist has labeled family resistance is in fact a lack of clarity on the therapist's part.

- *Collaboration:* Without collaboration between family members, as well as between the family and the therapist, there is no therapy. Collaboration is an active process in which each step in the treatment must be negotiated and agreed on. Sometimes family members change their minds in the midst of treatment. If not addressed, this can result in a breakdown in progress.

- *Family responsibility:* Therapists describe a sense of working too hard with some families. In such cases it is necessary to shift the balance of responsibility evenly between the therapist and the family. Ultimately, it is the family who must do the work that is necessary to reach their desired goals. It is the therapist's responsibility to facilitate an environment in which that change can take place.

- *Focus on the present:* When, in session after session, the same issues are discussed over and over again, therapists express frustration at getting nowhere with the family. These are telltale signs that the work is more focused on talking about than on acting on problems. The past is useful only to the extent that it affects today's functioning. Allowing families to continuously wallow in the unfortunate water that has gone under the bridge is not only unproductive but can be dangerous. Inadvertently, the therapist may be facilitating a sense of hopelessness in the family.

■ REFERENCES

Alves JW: Back to basics is good move when "stuck" in family therapy. The Brown University Family Therapy Letter, August 1992

Anderson C, Stewart S: Mastering Resistance: A Practical Guide to Family Therapy. New York, Guilford, l983

Bowen M: Family Therapy in Clinical Practice. New York, Jason Aronson, 1978

Haley J, Hoffman L. Techniques of Family Therapy. New York, Basic Books, 1967

Imber-Black E: Secrets in Families and Family Therapy. New York, Norton, 1993

Napier A, Whitaker C: The Family Crucible. New York, Harper and Row, 1978

Satir VM, Baldwin M: Satir Step by Step: A Guide to Creating Change in Families. Palo Alto, CA, Science and Behavior Books, 1983

10

FAMILY TREATMENT: GENERAL CONSIDERATIONS

In the following discussion, we consider more general features of marital and family treatment, namely, the participants, the setting, the scheduling of treatment, and the use of family therapy in combination with other treatment methods and helping agencies.

■ FAMILY PARTICIPANTS

In practice, it is often preferable to begin treatment by seeing the entire family together. The family can broadly be defined to include all persons living under the same roof; all those persons closely related to one another, even though they do not live together; or, even more broadly, all persons who are significant to the family, even though not related to them, such as friends, caregivers, or the social network.

Sometimes family therapy is carried out with the same therapist meeting with the whole family and with each family member individually. This is termed *concurrent family therapy* and is uncommon today. At other times two therapists who maintain some contact with each other, but who do not work jointly, may each see separately one or more members of a family in what is known as *collaborative family therapy*. *Conjoint family therapy* has been defined as family therapy in which the participants include at least two generations of a family, such as parents and children, plus the therapist, all meeting together. *Conjoint marital therapy* is limited to the two spouses plus the therapist meeting together.

The preferred model for family therapists is to see the whole family together for most of the sessions, occasionally having sessions with one of the subsystems (parents alone, siblings alone, father-son, etc.) as needed. Therapists who are interested in family-of-origin work also have some sessions with one of the spouses and their parents. Opinion is divided as to whether individual therapy with one or more members should be done while family therapy is in progress and whether the individual therapist should also be the family therapist. Concurrent individual therapy is sometimes done by a separate therapist, who preferably has some communication with the family therapist. In may cases, family therapy is suggested by the therapist of a child or spouse who then continues to treat his or her patient while family therapy continues.

Although it often seems desirable to meet with all family members, in actual practice this may be impossible or even contraindicated. For example, when discussing the sexual adjustment of the parents, the children should not be present. Often, too, the therapist is unable to include members because of illness, divorce, or death or because one or more family members temporarily or permanently refuses to participate. A decision must be made, either at the outset of treatment or after the evaluation, as to whether it is worthwhile and possible to continue working with the incomplete family. Hard-and-fast rules as to when it is worthwhile are not easy to give, but our bias is that if the pros and cons are about equal, it is better to give treatment a try even if the family is incomplete.

At times individuals feel uncomfortable talking about certain topics in front of the other family members. In such instances, the family therapist must use his or her judgment as to when individual interviewing might be indicated. This might be done, for example, with the goal of eventually bringing the material from the individual session to the entire family group. It must be recognized that there may be family secrets that cannot be productively shared with other family members and that should be kept private between an individual family member and the therapist. For example, one of the most complex current issues is whether children should be told that they are products of artificial insemination or other assisted reproductive techniques. Current thinking holds that the emotional problems for the family of not knowing or of having a secret are worse than dealing with it, but we have no real proof that this is the case. On this issue, too, no rigid guidelines can be established.

■ TIME, SCHEDULING, AND FEES

Most family therapists see a family once a week for 45–90 minutes. In outpatient settings, a minority of therapists see a family more than once a week. In inpatient settings, family sessions may be scheduled more frequently. The frequency of sessions is somewhat arbitrary; meeting less frequently may be strategically better for some families.

The decision as to the overall duration of treatment depends in part on the goals of treatment. On the average, family therapy is a short-term method as compared with individual or group psychotherapy or psychoanalysis. Other ground rules are as follows:

- Missed appointments should be rescheduled that week, if possible.
- When one member of the family is late in arriving at a session, the therapist may start the clock at the arranged time and proceed with whoever is present. The therapist can present the position of the absent member. On the other hand, in order to put pressure on everyone to come on time, many therapists do not start therapy until everyone has arrived.
- What can be done if one member of the family will not come to treatment? Often the resistance is not just from the member who will not come but also partly from the other members of the family, who covertly (or overtly) encourage such an absence. They may be unaware of their collusion, however, and often ask for help to get the reluctant member to participate. Therefore, one possibility is for the therapist to contact the absent member.
- Fees are usually set by time, that is, the length of the session, not by the number of members of the family present.

■ KEEPING A RECORD OF TREATMENT

Opinions differ as to the value of keeping written notes on the course of family treatment. Such a record may be useful in both monitoring goals and recording changes. A problem-oriented record, modified for families, provides a concise, overall picture of the identified patient and the family and outlines problems, goals, and strategies (Deming and Kimble 1975). Ongoing progress notes record significant family developments, enable measurement of goal achievement, and provide a record of treatment and modalities used for achieving these goals. Referrals to other agencies are also noted. Such a system has a distinct advantage over the traditional practice of keeping a separate record for each family member.

Many therapists focus on the process rather than the content of the sessions and therefore believe that there is no need to write down the facts of what goes on. Others prefer not to keep any records of treatment, to protect themselves against the possibility of being subpoenaed. We disagree, and our bias is to keep succinct and relevant records in all cases. We also believe that records are very helpful for both legal and training purposes.

Guidelines from the American Psychiatric Association are as follows:

> In family therapy, although it may be preferable to keep records on a family basis, it is usually more practical to keep them in one of the participant's individual charts, as most facilities maintain records in this manner. Since authorization from the patient named in the chart is generally sufficient for the release of information, care must be taken about information included about other family members. Whether or not the record is kept on an individual or a family basis, it may be wise to have all of the involved family members sign a statement at the beginning of therapy acknowledging that it will contain information about all of them and specifying which signatures or combination thereof will be required to authorize access to the chart or release information from it. In the event of substantial family change, such as divorce or a child's reaching majority, particular care should be exercised not to release information inappropriately. (American Psychiatric Association 1987, p. 1524)

■ FAMILY THERAPY IN COMBINATION WITH OTHER PSYCHOSOCIAL THERAPIES

At present, the differential effectiveness of family therapy alone compared with its use in combination with other therapies is just beginning to be studied. The use of family therapy in combination with somatic, individual, and group therapy has increased and is now common practice.

A minority of family therapists uses conjoint family therapy alone. All contacts are kept strictly within the joint family setting, and the therapist does not communicate, even by telephone, with individual family members. No other treatment, including individual therapy, is used. This is done to avoid any type of coalition derived from material shared by the therapist and any part of the family system.

It is becoming more common for the same therapist to employ individual psychotherapy sessions combined with family therapy. In this arrangement, the therapist has the advantage of knowing both the individual and the family. This combination, however, changes the nature of the therapy as follows:

1. The patient in individual therapy may feel that what he or she reveals in the one-to-one situation may in some way (either overtly or covertly) be communicated to the family by the therapist.
2. Family members may be reluctant to deal with sensitive issues in the conjoint sessions, preferring to reveal them in individual sessions.
3. Transference in individual sessions does not develop as fully, because patients can directly express their feelings about their families in the family therapy.

Items 1 and 2 must be dealt with directly; item 3 is not a major problem because in these situations the therapy is usually not transference based.

In addition to conjoint family treatment, individual therapy may be simultaneously carried out with only one patient or with both parents in separate sessions. In these cases, a colleague of the family therapist may conduct the individual therapy. It cannot be stressed too strongly that communication between therapists is necessary for effective collaborative treatment.

A major shift in the 1990s was marked by the notion of using different formats over different stages of therapy and periods of time. A common sequence of treatment is as follows. A couple presents with a sexual problem. Sexual therapy solves the problem. At this point, marital problems come to the fore. Marital therapy is then employed, and the marital relationship is improved. After this, one or both members of the couple may decide that they want to explore different aspects of their own growth and development; therefore, individual sessions or therapy are scheduled. Numerous variations on this concept are possible, and the important issue for the beginning therapist to understand is that this kind of sequencing is an increasing trend.

Sugarman (1986) describes some rules of thumb in making decisions about combined therapy, which are shown in Table 10–1. Table 10–2 lists contraindications to combining modalities.

TABLE 10–1. **Rules of thumb for combined therapies**

Combined therapy is useful if

It appears that different modalities would help significantly in different dimensions, such as the biological, social, and psychological

It appears that a given modality is either not helpful or of limited usefulness without an additional modality

There is significant motivation on the part of the individual or family to combine modalities

The modalities are synergistic and enhance each other

Source: Adapted from Sugarman 1986.

TABLE 10–2. **Contraindications to combining modalities**

The epistemological foundations of the various modalities are often based on contradictory assumptions. Because the goal of clinical work is to provide a coherent cognitive ordering of the world, combining modalities can at times be unproductively confusing for the patient system.

The additional time and money involved may be unnecessary. A single modality is often powerful enough to accomplish what is therapeutically necessary.

Different modalities can dilute the potential catharsis available for each separate therapeutic involvement. To the extent that there is meaning to the concept of psychic energy, it can be divided between the various modalities with not enough available in any one for the critical mass necessary to accomplish therapeutic work. This is similar to the concept in psychoanalytic thought of diluting the transference.

Individual treatment as a supplement to conjoint family therapy has also been carried out with one parent or a child. Individual sessions supplemented by conjoint sessions for all family members is an approach that is employed commonly in child psychiatric practice.

Family therapy may be prescribed in combination with group therapy and with behavioral therapy. It has been used in conjunction with hospitalization and partial hospitalization for one member (usually the identified patient) or for all members of the family in both inpatient and day hospital settings. It has also been used in conjunction with psychiatric medications and electroconvulsive therapy, which are used to control the identified patient's acute symptoms. In some situations, we have found that marital therapy was possible, and effective, only after one or both marital partners had been treated for depression (which predated the marriage) with antidepressants.

Family therapy has been prescribed as an adjunct to individual therapy. In these situations, it may be useful for diagnostic purposes to correct distorted perceptions and to shorten treatment.

■ FAMILY THERAPY IN COMBINATION WITH PHARMACOTHERAPY

Since 1970, new medications—such as selective serotonin reuptake inhibitors; atypical antipsychotics; and anticonvulsants for the treatment of schizophrenia, depression, mania, borderline disorders, and other Axis I disorders—have created the opportunity to improve the prognosis for patients and their families (Glick et al 1996). As medication has become more effective, is therapy still useful, and how? An important part of the answer is to combine psychotherapy and/or rehabilitation strategies, especially family intervention, with newer medication strategies (Glick et al. 1993).

Research suggests that, although pharmacotherapy may be the cornerstone of treatment for Axis I disorders, it should be combined with individual and family work for almost all patients, and with family therapy at some point in the treatment. Reasons for this include the following:

- Family dynamic issues or other stress may precipitate episodes, and therapy can help families prevent or cope with further stress.
- Persons with these disorders often have lost (or have never acquired) social skills, or the illness has created behavior patterns that make these persons averse to their support systems, including, and especially, the family.
- The illness has powerful effects on family life, and the entire family needs to cope with this fact together.
- An ongoing relationship with the family therapist not only improves medication compliance but also provides continuous support during times when the person may not be on medication and provides a critical social support for persons dealing with what in many cases are chronic and potentially lifelong issues.

A modest number of controlled studies suggest that medication and family intervention are synergistic. Each covers different domains—medication decreases certain symptom clusters, such as hallucinations and delusions, and family intervention improves interpersonal skills and relationships. By extension, it is assumed that both of these treatments improve compliance. The obvious next questions that remain to be answered are "Which diagnoses need which combination of therapies? In which sequence? In what doses?"

Practical Guidelines

1. *Diagnosis:*   The therapist should be sure to make a DSM-IV-TR (American Psychiatric Association 2000) diagnosis, a family systems diagnosis, and an individual formulation of dynamics. Without a diagnostic map, the appropriate drug will not pre- scribed. So too, without a map of the family system dynamics, the clinician will be lost in the complexity of family issues.

2. *Goals:*   The therapist should set target symptoms for all mo- dalities. The issue here is to determine which symptoms are re- sponsive to medication and which are responsive to individual or family interventions. Without this delineation of target symptoms, it is impossible to know which treatment (or combi- nation) is effective.

3. *Untoward effects:*   The therapist should be aware of the side effects of drug therapy and of family and/or individual psycho- therapy, as well as their interaction. For example, increasing medications may allow the identified patient to be able to dis- cuss issues that were previously too emotionally charged for careful family discussion. Needless to say, untoward effects must be monitored at each session. For example, neuroleptic medication may create side effects (like sedation and dyspho- ria) that not only are unpleasant to the patient but may also de- crease the ability to socialize inside and outside of the family.

   In some situations, a patient, with or without the family, may use the improvement resulting from medication to avoid ex- ploring relevant family issues. Still, the family therapist should not avoid prescribing medications when necessary.

4. *For whom is combined family and/or individual treatment and medication not indicated?*   Obviously this combination is not

for everyone. We believe in the principle of therapeutic parsimony: If one modality is effective, do not add a second. To be explicit, for some clinical situations, we start with family therapy; for others, medication. In still others, we start both simultaneously and may withdraw one (or both) modalities over time. Family therapy may be the right modality at the right time. At the very least, putting aside the power of a family intervention by itself, the family systems approach is a very efficacious way to increase compliance.

The next issue is to effectively and efficiently sequence the modalities. Usually, as a first step, a working therapeutic alliance must be established. Only after this has been done should medication be prescribed. Simultaneously, if appropriate, the family should be referred to an appropriate consumer group, such as the National Alliance for the Mentally Ill, the National Depressive and Manic-Depressive Association, or Alcoholics Anonymous. Next, psychoeducation for the patient (if he or she is cognitively able) and the family is a crucial early step. This consists of the systematic administration over time of information about symptoms and signs, diagnosis, treatment, and prognosis. Individual supportive therapy and/or family supportive interventions are then made, and only later are dynamic individual or systemic family models used. Later, depending on response, rehabilitation is added to the equation.

The Medication Alliance

By way of comparison with the alliance in family therapy, we describe here what has been called the *pharmacotherapeutic alliance*. This alliance can be defined as the manner in which active efforts are made by the physician to enlist and involve the patient in a collaboration around the use of medication. The physician must be flexible in his or her stance, focus on medication issues, and acknowledge that a certain amount of uncertainty accompanies the treatment process. The physician must work to establish and maintain an alliance with the patient. This process includes shared inquiry, shared goals, and mutual participation, both in the experience and in the observation of the process of using medication.

Family Intervention

We now turn to the family intervention part of the equation. Lam (1991) described the following seven components of effective family approaches to schizophrenia, but each of these can be adapted to most Axis I and Axis II disorders:

1. A positive approach and genuine working relationship between the therapist and family
2. The provision of family therapy in a stable, structured format with the availability of additional contacts with therapists if necessary
3. A focus on improving stress and coping in the here and now rather than dwelling on the past
4. Encouragement of respect for interpersonal boundaries within the family
5. The provision of information about the biological nature of the illness in order to reduce blaming of the patient and family guilt
6. The use of behavioral techniques, such as breaking down goals into manageable steps
7. Improving communication among family members

The essence of the family intervention when combined with medication is as follows:

- Education about the disorder—its signs and symptoms, causes, and biological as well as psychosocial treatments
- Communication skills training to improve the quality of family transactions and reduce family tension
- Problem-solving skills training for managing family- and/or illness-related conflicts and reducing family burden
- Resolution of dynamic and systems issues created by the disorder

The essence of the pharmacological intervention when combined with the family intervention is to normalize the illness (as with lithium in bipolar disorder) and suppress symptoms in the individual. To summarize, family therapy somewhat paradoxically can ultimately and indirectly promote medication compliance, whereas medication can improve interpersonal function and compliance with family therapy.

■ REFERENCES

American Psychiatric Association, Committee on Confidentiality: Guidelines on confidentiality. Am J Psychiatry 144:1522–1526, 1987

American Psychiatric Association: Diagnostic and Statistical Manual of Mental Disorders, 4th Edition, Text Revision. Washington, DC, American Psychiatric Association, 2000

Deming B, Kimble JJ: Adapting the individual problem-oriented record for use with families. Hosp Community Psychiatry 26:334–335, 1975

Glick ID, Clarkin JF, Goldsmith SJ: Combining medication with family psychotherapy, in the American Psychiatric Press Review of Psychiatry, Vol. 12. Edited by Oldham JH, Riba MB, Tasman A. Washington, DC, American Psychiatric Association, 1993, pp 585–610

Glick ID, Lecrubier Y, Montgomery S, et al: Efficacious and safe psychotropics not available in the United States. Psychiatr Ann 26:354–361, 1996

Lam DH: Psychosocial family intervention in schizophrenia: a review of empirical studies. Psychol Med 21:423–441, 1991

Sugarman S (ed): Interface of Individual and Family Therapy: Family Therapy Collection. Rockville, MD, Aspen, 1986

11

DYSFUNCTIONAL COUPLES
AND COUPLES THERAPY

■ MARITAL DIFFICULTIES, PROBLEMS, AND DYSFUNCTION

Some periods of dysfunction are inevitable in any long-term relationship. The burdens of sharing intimate, social, and parenting roles mean that people will inevitably clash over some aspects of life. It is common for marriages to undergo periodic stages of crisis and reorganization. Problems occur when couples lose faith in the marriage or lose a sense of respect and warmth for each other. Partners who have had poor role models, who had a childhood of loss and violence, or who are poorly suited to each other by style or inclination will have increasing problems over time.

Individuals come to marriage with the legacy of several generations of their family of origin, in addition to the beliefs and role models of their parents. This means they carry with them firm ideas about what marriage should be like, how men and women should behave, and what behaviors signify love and respect. From a developmental point of view, there remain unresolved needs and demands left from childhood that are invested with deeply ambivalent feelings of love and hate.

In the process of mate selection, the partner is attractive partly because he or she promises rediscovery of an important lost aspect of the subject's own personality, or because he or she offers the chance to redo an unfinished conflict with a parent. When the couple join, they make a marital contract in which they assume that each partner will do certain things (Sager 1976). Some of these ideas are conscious and shared ("You will care for the children, and I will work"), some are not shared, and some are secret even from the self. For example, a person may marry to get away from home or may believe that, as long as he or she acts like a good child, the spouse will act like a good parent. Mate selection, of course, is also determined by less dynamic reasons, such as physical attractiveness, family demands, financial considerations, timing, and luck.

Treatment for the couple involves increasing the intensity of the affective bonds and repairing their inevitable disruption. Each partner must have someone who listens to his or her experience (i.e., the narrative) and helps to sort it out. Lewis (1998) said that "[t]he prerequisites include a genuine and reciprocal liking for each other, mutual respect, a two-way valuing and affirmation" (p. 584). That author also suggests that couples need to learn conflict management mechanisms, including techniques to prevent isolation. Couple communication, that is, how people talk to each other, can alter relationships. To improve disconnections, the therapist must teach intimate communication, focusing on how to explore difficult issues and increase empathy.

The strongest predictor of overall life satisfaction is the quality of a person's central relationship. In addition, a "good and stable relationship buffers against the genetic vulnerabilities to both medical and psychiatric disorder" (J.M. Lewis, personal communication, May 1998).

Dynamic Point of View

Many individuals who need assistance with marital conflict seem to have a rigidity in their personalities that forces them to deny or to be blind to the existence of certain aspects of themselves. If they are confronted with a similar aspect of the partner's personality, it is ignored or rejected. Such people may project onto the partner aspects of their own personality with which they are uncomfortable. They are therefore prevented from seeing the problem clearly or seeking alternative solutions. Often third parties are used to interfere and deflect conflict between the partners.

Gender differences in needs and communication often make marital problems more complex. Men are more likely to wish for deference, to wish to deal with their problems by themselves before talking about them, and to see sex as a way of solving problems. Women are more likely to wish for verbal intimacy and task equality, to want to deal with problems by discussion and "feeling talk" first rather than only discuss solutions, and to see sex as possible only after problems are solved. Women tend to experience the emotional burden of the relationship as falling on them. Men tend to see themselves as more responsible for the family's finances, even when the wife is working. Therefore, in a fairly large number of cases, the woman finds herself emotionally pursuing and sexually unhappy, whereas the man finds himself criticized for his need to be less emotional, even though he has been trained to control most of his feelings. (Obviously, not all individuals fit these gender stereotypes.)

As a couple struggles over different ways of behaving or different and ambivalent needs, each sees the other as unhelpful or bad and begins to become angry. This escalates into a cycle of distress.

Behavioral Point of View

From a behavioral point of view, distressed couples engage in fewer rewarding exchanges and more punishing exchanges than do nondistressed couples. Distressed couples are more likely to reciprocate each other's use of negative reinforcement and to eventually go on the offensive by increasing the level of punishment, regardless of the stimuli. Distressed couples are also likely to attempt to control the behavior of one another through negative communication and the withholding of positive communication. They strive for behavior change in the other by aversive control tactics, that is, by strategically presenting punishment and withholding rewards.

Systems Point of View

From a systems point of view, the solution becomes the problem—that is, more aversive control (silence or attack) produces more aversive behavior in the spouse instead of the longed-for connection. In addition, triangles form to deflect conflict, so that children, friends, parents, or lovers are drawn into the marital conflict.

Psychiatric Illness Point of View

Having a spouse with a serious Axis I disorder, such as anxiety disorder, mood disorder, or substance abuse, strains the marital relationship. The marital interaction before, during, and after the onset of symptoms in the spouse is influenced by numerous factors and is quite variant across dyads. It is false to assume that in all cases the interaction between the spouses brought on, or caused, or even helped to trigger the mental disorder and symptoms in the other. Whatever the symptoms in one spouse, their relationship to the marital interaction exists on a continuum and can take any one of the following forms:

- The marital interaction neither causes the symptoms nor stresses the psychologically vulnerable spouse.
- The marital interaction does not stress the vulnerable individual, but after the onset of symptoms, the marital interaction declines and becomes dysfunctional, thus causing greater distress.
- The marital interaction acts as a stressor that contributes to the onset of symptoms in a vulnerable spouse.
- The symptoms can be explained totally as under the control and function of the interactional patterns between the spouses.

The therapist meeting a new couple can therefore entertain a range of different ideas that may help to illuminate and explain their distressing circumstances.

■ COUPLES/MARITAL THERAPY

Definition

Couples therapy can be defined as a format of intervention involving both members of a dyad in which the focus of the intervention is the dysfunctional and displeasing interactional patterns of the couple. Couples or marital therapy focuses on the dyad and its intimate emotional and sexual aspects, whereas family therapy usually focuses on issues involving the behavior of a child or adolescent and the interactions between parents and children. In family therapy, one can discern triangles involving various family members, whereas in couples or marital work, triangles in the family must be inferred and triangulation in the here-and-now interaction must involve the therapist (because there are only two family members present). Marital therapy sessions are usually attended by only the spouses, although the children may be invited during the initial assessment or later for specific issues.

Couples therapy is distinguished by the peer relationship of the participants, the ever-present questions of commitment, and a need to carefully attend to gender issues. In general, even if therapy is behaviorally focused, it must attend particularly to the feeling level, having as its goal creating more positive feelings between the partners as well as more reasonable behavior.

The Issue of Commitment—The Problem of Affairs

Assessing a couple's motivation becomes more complex when one spouse expresses commitment to the relationship at the beginning of therapy but is secretly carrying on an affair and plans to leave the relationship once the final attempt at therapy requested by the spouse is completed. Although it was once thought that one partner could not help knowing about the other's affair, further experience has taught us that, with a fairly emotionally distant marriage in which there is still a great deal of trust, many things can be kept secret by a determined person. Often marital therapy is precipitated by the partner discovering the affair. In this case it is no longer secret, but the marriage is profoundly altered.

Many therapists will not proceed with marital treatment unless a spouse who is actively engaged in an extramarital situation terminates the affair immediately. Some will proceed with treatment if the affair is known to the partner, at least for a time while the couple decides what to do next. It is believed impossible to conduct effective couples therapy when one spouse and the therapist are keeping an affair secret from the other spouse. It is probably also impossible for a spouse who is having an affair to have the energy necessary to work on the marriage, although the therapist may be able to persuade the wandering spouse to give up the affair and return to the marriage at least long enough for a reasonable attempt.

Evaluation of Partners

With the obvious modification of focusing mainly on the marital dyad, the outline for family evaluation (see Chapter 4) can be used for the evaluation of a marital pair seeking assistance with their troubled relationship. This involves obtaining data on the current point in the family and marital life cycle, why the couple come for assistance at this time, and each of their views of the marital problem. In formulating the marital difficulty, the evaluator will want to summarize his or her thoughts around the couple's communication, problem solving, roles, affective expression and involvement, and behavioral expression, especially in sexual and aggressive areas. The clinician will also want to evaluate gender roles, cultural and racial issues, and power inequities in terms of gender, class, age, or financial status. It is critical to ask about alcohol, health and reproductive issues, and violence. Even if the partners do not mention the children as a problem, it is wise to spend some time developing a sense of how the children are doing, whether there are favorites or problems, and whether they are being pulled into marital conflicts. The clinician should also ascertain whether there is a diagnosable condition, especially an Axis I disorder, in either or both partners.

Several areas embedded in the above general categories deserve special evaluation attention. These include each spouse's commitment to the marital union and the sexual expression of this commitment or lack thereof. Both conjoint and individual assessment interviews with each of the partners may be needed. Infidelity or serious questions about commitment changes the character of the couple's therapy from how the couple manage to whether the couple will stay together. It is possible, however, to ask the couple to drop the affair or divorce plans for a specified period, assume they are in the marriage to stay, and try to change it.

The complicated issue of how to obtain information about the degree of commitment and ongoing marital affairs, as well as other private information, can be handled in various ways. We recommend that, as a part of the marital evaluation, the therapist hold one individual session with each partner after the first or second conjoint session. These sessions are usually considered confidential. However, the therapist may reserve the right not to continue treatment unless the spouse gives the partner relevant information, such as the existence of an ongoing affair or HIV-positive status. The therapist may give the partner a few weeks or an extra session to plan for this disclosure but is not obligated to conduct therapy in situations where holding the secret is untenable. Although some therapists prefer not to know certain secrets, we believe that it is futile to proceed with therapy in the face of an overwhelming secret as though it did not exist. If a matter such as incest, violence, or alcohol abuse is known to the couple but is kept secret from the therapist, it is also best that the therapist hear it early, in private session, and find a way to bring it into the couples work.

It is often difficult to determine whether couples therapy is the treatment of choice and whether other therapy should be given, either concurrently or sequentially. For example, a member of the couple may need concurrent medication or may be having enough other problems with work, parents, or personality difficulties that he or she has no energy left for couples work. In general, couples who come in for therapy together should be given evaluation, support, and education, as well as a clear picture of how the couples issues connect with the individual issues. If appropriate, partners may be referred for concurrent individual therapy or may be asked to have individual therapy first and return for couples work later. In other cases, the couple's therapist may do individual work concurrently or within the dyad. Some recommend against having the same therapist do individual work with only one partner and then do the couples work, because the therapist tends to become more bonded to the person with whom they do the individual work. Others believe that this disadvantage is outweighed by having one therapist know the system's issues and therefore doing both the individual and the marital therapy.

Couples in which there has been active violence are not candidates for couples work unless the couple is holding to a clear contract that no violence will occur. Violent men usually need their own therapy as well; group treatment has proven effective in many cases. In many cases, both partners are violent.

Goals

The mediating goals of couples therapy, which involve a mix of theoretical frameworks, include specification of the interactional problems, recognition of mutual contribution to the problems, clarification of marital boundaries, clarification and specification of each spouse's needs and desires in the relationship, increased communication skills, decreased coercion and blame, increased differentiation, and resolution of marital transference distortions. Final goals of the marital intervention may involve resolution of presenting problems, reduction of symptoms, increased intimacy, increased role flexibility and adaptability, toleration of differences, improved psychosexual functioning, balance of power, clear communication, resolution of conflictual interaction, and improved relationships with children and families of origin (Gurman 1981).

Couples therapy need not be, but is often, conceived of as a relatively brief therapy, usually consisting of meetings on a once-weekly basis and having a focus on the marital interaction. There are times when bringing in one or both spouse's parents or children may be beneficial for cutting through issues that are affecting the marriage (Framo 1981). The major indication for marital intervention is the presence of marital conflict contributed to by both parties, but indications may also include symptomatic behavior, such as depression or agoraphobia, in one spouse. Marital treatment is contraindicated, even when the above conditions are present, when the two parties would use treatment disclosures to injure the other.

If the couples therapy seems to consistently escalate conflict, then the goals should be reevaluated.

Strategies and Techniques of Intervention

Like family therapy in general, couples therapy uses strategies for imparting new information, opening up new and expanded individual and marital experiences, psychodynamic strategies for individual and interactional insight, communication and problem-solving strategies, and strategies for restructuring the repetitive interactions between the spouses. We advocate an integrative marital therapy model that uses psychodynamic, behavioral, and structural-strategic strategies of intervention.

A Model for Intervention Based on Patterns of Interaction

Although couples may show conflict over specific content issues, such as handling finances, allocating time to each other, and reconciling individual and family needs, the therapist is usually confronted with redundant patterns of interaction that are likely to become the focus of treatment. For example, in one couple, the wife tries to explain something important to her husband about her need to feel emotionally connected to him; he reacts negatively to her tone of voice (saying he feels criticized) and retreats; she responds by suggesting that he is simply pushing her away and feels unloved; and so on. This pattern of pursuit-withdrawal might well occupy the attention of the therapist, who may notice that it occurs irrespective of the particular topic of conversation.

Other patterns involve either complementarity or symmetry in relationships. In complementary relationships, the overfunctioning of one member may invite the underfunctioning of the other (e.g., responsible-irresponsible, nurse-patient). Because the pattern is presumed to be reciprocal, the description can be punctuated in the opposite form just as correctly; that is, the underfunctioning of one invites the overfunctioning of the other. In symmetrical relationships, the therapist often encounters a power struggle in which each member is engaged in asserting his or her own position in order to gain the one-up position or to avoid feeling one-down. It is essential that gender arrangements be examined in relation to both the complementary and the symmetrical roles that men and women find themselves enacting with each other.

Data suggest that the diagnosis and symptom picture of the spouse and the characteristics of the other spouse stand in complex relationship to the issues in the marital interaction and should, therefore, influence the planning of intervention, that is, the goals. For example, if one spouse has a nonendogenous, unipolar depression with no clear precipitating stressful life events, the marital interaction could be a chronic stressor and contributor to the condition. Marital therapy in this situation could well be a preferred mode of intervention. On the other hand, if the spouse has a bipolar illness, manic episode, and the marital interaction has been good before the episode, psychoeducational intervention with the couple may be in order, with little or no attention to the ongoing marital interaction.

Sometimes, couples present with chronic histories of unresolved and unrelenting conflict. Other couples are in a state of transition, perhaps moving from the initial expansion stage of their marriage to the inevitable crisis related to the reevaluation of the contraction stage. In either case, clarifying the couple's process—their recurring patterns of behavior—represents the starting place for couples therapy.

Individual Models

Once the therapist understands the couple's specific problem and has defined it as a pattern that each member contributes to maintaining, the goals is to determine what constrains the couple from making the needed changes. It can generally be assumed that patterns are developed from the members' individual models of marriage learned in their families and in prior relationships and by their own traditions of relating to one another as a couple. In considering historical models, the therapist might suppose that each member of a couple brings his or her own images or model of how intimate relationships should proceed. The therapist can collect and organize historical data through the use of a genogram, the three-generational family tree depicting the family's patterns regarding either specific problems or general family functioning. The genogram technique suggests possible connections between present family events and past experiences that family members have shared (e.g., regarding the management of serious illnesses, losses, and other critical transitions), thereby placing the presenting problem in a historical context (McGoldrick and Gerson 1985; Shorter 1977). Constructing a genogram early on in treatment can provide a wealth of data that frequently offers clues about pressures, expectations, and hopes regarding the marriage. This pictorial way of gathering a history allows each member of the couple to learn about the beliefs or themes that characterize his or her family background.

The therapist can then try to help the couple understand how their own preferred patterns (which may, in fact, relate to earlier family models) have limited their ability to flexibly adapt and change. The predictability with which they will respond to unmet needs and disappointments can be supportively pointed out so that each member of the couple begins to understand the specific ways in which they enact the same process over and over again. If this is the only process the couple knows, they may become despondent on recognizing the limitations of their emotional-behavioral repertoire. However, with support and active interventions, the couples therapist can begin to help the couple to conduct experiments with each other that are aimed at expanding their ways of relating to each other.

Strategies for Change

Although each school of couples and family treatment advocates its own emphasis on particular aspects of the change process (e.g., changing couples' beliefs or cognitions, changing behavioral sequences, increasing differentiation, expanding emotional awareness), some relatively enduring characteristics of most marital therapies can be identified.

The focus should be primarily on the interpersonal distortions between the partners, and not on the couple-therapist transference. However, negative transference distortions toward the therapist must be addressed quickly and overtly.

There are three strategies in this focused, active treatment of marital discord:

1. The therapist interrupts collusive processes between the spouses. The interaction may involve either spouse failing to perceive positive or negative aspects of the other that are clear to an outsider (e.g., generosity or cruelty) or either spouse behaving in a way that is aimed at protecting the other from experiences that are inconsistent with that spouse's self-perception (e.g., a husband who works part-time views himself as breadwinner, but his wife, who works full-time, manages the checkbook to shield her husband from the reality of their income and finances).
2. The therapist links individual experience, including past experience and inner thoughts, to the marital relationship.
3. The therapist creates and assigns tasks that are constructed to 1) encourage each partner to differentiate between the impact of the other's behavior versus the other's intent, 2) bring into awareness the concrete behavior of the partner that contradicts (anachronistic) past perceptions of that partner, and 3) encourage each partner to acknowledge his or her own behavior changes that are incompatible with the maladaptive ways in which each has seen himself or herself and has been seen by the marital partner. These exercises also help to reconstruct the couple's narrative to make it more positive.

The last (item 3) is most important. In fact, in the initial stage of marital treatment, we ask that both partners focus on what they want to change in themselves, not how they want the spouse to be different.

Returning to the integrative marital therapy model mentioned earlier, this model assumes that effective marital treatment does not artificially dichotomize individual and relationship change, and thus focuses on both. The model assumes that not all the behaviors of one partner are under the interactional control of the other, and that even behavior with an obvious relationship to the marital interaction is not completely under relational control. Furthermore, Gurman (1981) asserts that adoption of a systems perspective does not preclude attention to unconscious aspects of experience. In fact, self-perceptions are the mechanisms that power the behavior—maintaining aspects of interpersonal reinforcement.

In this integrative model, the goals of assessment are to evaluate three related domains: 1) the functional relationships between the antecedents and consequences of discrete interactional sequences; 2) the recurrent patterns of interaction, including their implicit rules; and 3) each spouse's individual schemata for intimate relationships. In the initial stage, alliances must be developed early between the therapist and each marital partner as the therapist offers empathy, warmth, and understanding. The therapist must also ally with the couple as a whole and learn their shared language as well as their different problem-solving styles and attitudes.

Behavioral techniques, including giving between-session homework, in-session tasks, communication skills, and problem-solving training, can facilitate the process of helping marital partners reintegrate denied aspects of themselves and of each other. However, the focus is not on behavioral change alone, as overt behavior is seen as reflecting the interlocking feelings and perceptions of each spouse. Ideally, the process of treatment should be one in which the partners can consider what they want to change in themselves as opposed to how they want the other spouse to be different; safely explore new beliefs, feelings, and behaviors; and experiment with new patterns of interaction that are unfamiliar and even anxiety provoking.

■ REFERENCES

Framo JL: The integration of marital therapy with family of origin sessions, in Handbook of Family Therapy. Edited by Gurman AS, Kninskern DP. New York, Brunner/Mazel, 1981, pp 133–158

Gurman A: Integrative marital therapy: toward the development of an interpersonal approach, in Forms of Brief Therapy. Edited by Budman S. New York, Guilford, 1981, pp 415–457

Lewis JM: For better or worse: interpersonal relationships and individual outcome. Am J Psychiatry 155:582–589, 1998

McGoldrick M, Gerson R: Genograms in Family Assessment. New York, Norton, 1985

Sager C: Marriage Contracts and Couple Therapy: Hidden Forces in Intimate Relationships. New York, Brunner/Mazel, 1976

Shorter E: The Making of the Modern Family. New York, Basic Books, 1977

12

MARITAL AND SEX THERAPY

It has been estimated that 50% of American marriages have some sexual problems. These can be divided into *difficulties* (such as an inability to agree on frequency), which are clearly dyadic issues, and *dysfunctions*, which are specific problems with desire, arousal, and orgasm, as listed in DSM-IV-TR (American Psychiatric Association 2000). Dysfunctions may be organically or psychologically based and may be lifelong or acquired, generalized or situational. They may be deeply embedded in relational power or intimacy struggles, or may be the only problem in an otherwise well-functioning relationship. Although most family therapists have believed that there is no uninvolved partner when one member of a couple presents with sexual dysfunction, this is different from saying that the relationship itself is the cause of the dysfunction. The job of the family therapist is to ascertain, as well as possible, the etiology of the problem and to choose the most effective therapy, whether medical, individual, or relational.

■ DIAGNOSIS: SYSTEMS ISSUES

Sexual dysfunction or dissatisfaction is seldom caused by a psychiatric disorder (although depression and anxiety may often decrease sexual desire). It is commonly caused by ignorance of sexual anatomy and physiology, negative attitudes and self-defeating behavior, anger, power or intimacy issues with the partners, or medical/physiological problems. Male erection problems are proving increasingly amenable to medical forms of treatment. It is also important to remember that people vary enormously in the importance they place on the sexual, or erotic, in their lives. For example, in the book *The Social Organization of Sexuality* (Laumann et al. 1994), about a third of the people surveyed reported having sex at least twice a week, about a third a few times a month, and the rest a few times a year or not at all. In general, when sex is not part of a marriage over a long period, the relationship has less vitality and life. However, even well-functioning marriages may have periods in which sexuality is much less a part of the couple's lives (such as after the birth of a first child or during a family crisis). Different people have vastly different tolerance for such periods.

■ SOME PARAMETERS OF SEXUAL FUNCTION

Healthy sexual functioning can be thought of as resulting from relatively nonconflicted and self-confident attitudes about sex and the belief that the partner is pleased by one's performance. Conversely, when either partner has doubts about his or her sexual abilities or ability to please the other, his or her sexual performance may suffer. This self-absorption and anxiety characteristically produce a decrease in sexual performance and enjoyment and can lead to impotence and orgasmic difficulties. Couple and individual difficulties of various sorts might then follow. A vicious circle may be activated as worries are increased, leading to increasingly poor sexual performance.

Because sex is a way for each person to become vulnerable to the other, it is difficult to have sex when one is angry or not in a mood to be close (although some people can block out other feelings and keep the sexual area separate). In addition, people who feel abused, mistreated, or ignored in a relationship are less likely to want to please the other. For some who feel that they have no voice in the relationship, lack of desire is sometimes the only way they feel able to manifest displeasure.

Couples who continue in marital or individual treatment for long periods can resolve some of their marital problems but may still experience specific sexual difficulties in their marriage. It is also true that specific sexual problems may be dramatically reversed after relatively brief periods of sex therapy, even though such problems may have proven intractable after long periods of more customary psychotherapy. However, sexual functioning that is suffering because the partners do not want to be close is not likely to respond to sex therapy unless other issues are also addressed.

Usually when a marital couple has a generally satisfactory relationship, any minor sexual problems may be only temporary. The resolution of sexual problems in a relationship, however, will not inevitably produce positive effects in other facets of a relationship as well.

Marital and sexual problems interact in various ways:

- *The sexual dysfunction produces or contributes to secondary marital discord.* Specific strategies focused on the sexual dysfunctions are usually considered the treatment of choice in these situations, especially if the same sexual dysfunction occurred in other relationships.
- *The sexual dysfunction is secondary to marital discord.* In such situations, general strategies of marital treatment might be considered the treatment of choice. If the marital relationship is not too severely disrupted, a trial of sex therapy might be attempted because a relatively rapid relief of symptoms could produce beneficial effects on the couple's interest in pursuing other marital issues.
- *Marital discord co-occurs with sexual problems.* This situation would probably not be amenable to sex therapy because of the partners' hostility to each other. Marital therapy would usually be attempted first and later attention given to sexual dysfunction.
- *Sexual dysfunction occurs without marital discord.* This case might be found in instances where one partner's medical illness has affected his or her sexual functioning, forcing the couple to learn new ways to manage the change. Another example might be when one partner has had a history of sexual abuse or a sexual

assault that creates anxiety related to the sexual experience. Although individual therapy can be helpful in both of these cases, couples therapy can be especially useful in creating a safe place to address painful feelings and anxious expectations and to provide education and guidance for couples undergoing these transitions.

■ ASSESSMENT OF SEXUAL DISORDER

The therapist should conduct a careful evaluation of the couple's total interactions, as well as a physical assessment when dysfunction is present. When it appears that the basic marriage is a sound one but that the couple is experiencing specific sexual difficulties (which may also lead to various secondary marital consequences), the primary focus might be sex therapy per se. In many cases, however, specific sex therapy cannot be carried out until the relationship between the two partners has been improved in other respects; indeed, the sexual problems may clearly be an outgrowth of the marital difficulties. When marital problems are taken care of, the sexual problems may be readily resolved. It may be difficult to disentangle marital from sexual problems or to decide which came first. The priorities for therapy may not always be clear.

DSM-IV-TR recognizes the following as sexual dysfunctions:

- *Sexual desire disorders:*   Hypoactive sexual desire disorder, sexual aversion disorder.
- *Sexual arousal disorders:*   Female sexual arousal disorder, male erectile disorder.
- *Orgasmic disorders:*   Female orgasmic disorder, male orgasmic disorder, premature ejaculation.
- *Sexual pain disorders:*   Dyspareunia (not due to a general medical condition), vaginismus (not due to a general medical condition), male or female dyspareunia (due to a general medical condition), and substance-induced sexual dysfunction with sexual pain. Disorders are coded separately if they are due to a general medical condition or are substance induced.

Many people have more than one dysfunction (for example, hypoactive sexual desire disorder plus orgasmic disorder), and frequently each member of a couple has a dysfunction, for example, premature ejaculation in the man and hypoactive desire in the woman. It is important to understand the sequencing of the onset of the dysfunctions to see how they influence each other. As we have said, many sexual problems are not dysfunctions but are relationally based dissatisfactions.

Specific techniques have been devised for eliciting a sexual history and for evaluating sexual functioning. The marital therapist should become familiar with these ideas and obtain experience in their use. A systemic assessment of sexual difficulties includes, at the minimum, the elements listed in Table 12–1.

A thorough discussion of assessment techniques for each specific sexual problem can be found in *Principles and Practice of Sex Therapy* (Leiblum and Rosen 1989). A sexual genogram is useful for those interested in family-of-origin work (Berman and Hof 1987).

In addition, in couples where there is any possibility that the problems may have an organic component, it is crucial to insist on a medical workup. This is particularly key for men, for whom small physiological changes in potency may produce anxiety that exacerbates the problem.

The taking of an intimate sexual history of husband and wife should, of course, be conducted with the couple without children present. The process of taking a sexual history should be handled with care and regard for each person's level of comfort. One should not use terms that would be offensive or uncomfortable for either the therapist or the couple. At the same time, care must be taken to avoid using bland generalities that fail to elicit little specific sexual information. Frankness is encouraged, and when there is vagueness, the therapist should follow up with more specific questions.

Taking a sexual history of lesbian and gay couples may be particularly difficult for a heterosexual therapist, either because of discomfort with homosexuality or lack of knowledge of homosexual norms and mores. In addition, the couple may have a wider or dif-

---

TABLE 12–1. **Assessment of sexual problems**

I. Definition of the problem
    A. How does the couple describe the problem? What are their theories about its etiology? How do they generally relate to their sexuality, as reflected in their language, attitudes toward sexuality, comfort level, and permission system?
    B. How is the problem a problem for them? What is the function of the problem in their relationship system? Is the relationship problem the central problem? Why now?

II. Relationship history
    A. Current partner
    B. Previous relationship history
    C. Psychosexual history, including information about early childhood experiences, nature of sexual encounters prior to the relationship, sexual orientation, feelings about masculinity and femininity
    D. Description of current sexual functioning, focusing on conditions for satisfactory sex, positive behaviors, specific technique, and so on. Who initiates sex, who leads, or do both? How does the couple's sexual pattern of intimacy and control reflect or compensate for other aspects of their relationship?

III. Developmental life cycle issues (births, deaths, transitions)

IV. Medical history, focusing on current physical status, medications, and present medical care, especially endocrine, vascular, metabolic

V. Goals (patients' and therapist's viewpoints): the task is to examine whether goals are realistic and what previously attempted solutions have yielded.

Source. Reprinted from Glick ID, Berman EM, Clarkin JF, et al: *Marital and Family Therapy*, 4th Edition, 2000, p. 403. Copyright 2000, American Psychiatric Press, Inc. Used with permission.

ferent set of sexual practices than the therapist is used to (of course, this may be true with heterosexual couples as well). The therapist has the options of educating himself or herself about homosexual sexuality (the number of books available in mainstream bookstores about gay and lesbian life has risen dramatically in the last few years) and/or asking the couple about their own and other common practices. A therapist who is very anxious in this situation must decide when he or she is not an effective therapist and should refer to a colleague. Gay and lesbian couples may present with any of the dysfunctions or dissatisfactions of heterosexual couples.

■ TREATMENT

The form of treatment for psychosexual disorders developed by Masters and Johnson (1966) consisted of a thorough assessment of the partners and the relationship, education about sexual functioning, and a series of behavioral exercises. The model was based on three fundamental postulates: 1) a parallel sequence of physiological and subjective arousal in both sexes; 2) the primacy of psychogenic factors, particularly learning deficits and performance anxiety; and 3) the amenability of most sexual disorders to a brief, problem-focused treatment approach—that is, a sensate focus. These sensate focus exercises were designed predominantly for behavioral desensitization but also functioned to teach the partners about their own and each other's sexual desires and served to elicit awareness of relationship problems. In these exercises, the couple pleasures each other, alternating in the role of giver and receiver, first in nongenital areas, then genitally, then with intercourse. In the traditional form, intercourse is prohibited during the early stages to remove performance anxiety. There are also specific exercises for each of the sexual dysfunctions. (For a complete description of these exercises, we recommend the works of Kaplan [1995], Lo-Piccolo and Stock [1996], and Zilbergeld [1992].) This method works best when there is ignorance, shame, or specific dysfunction such as premature ejaculation. They are difficult to complete if the couple feels angry or unloving toward each other.

Recent writers in the field, particularly Schnarch (1997), have focused on cognitive/emotional issues in sexuality, particularly the meanings attached to a particular act and the level of intimacy involved. Now that sex researchers have learned a great deal about the more mechanical and organic issues related to arousal and orgasm, it is important to rethink other aspects of sex, such as eroticism, passion, mystery, and dominance and submission, which make the act itself meaningful. This is particularly true in areas of sexual boredom or situational lack of desire. These therapists do not use rigidly staged exercises but focus on the couple's relatedness during sex; they may, however, suggest specific homework to help a couple focus on a particular aspect of their sexuality.

Although not mentioned in DSM-IV-TR, the question of sexual compulsions or addictions may be seen in couples. In these cases, one partner's unceasing compulsion to think about, talk about, and have sex may be very wearing to the other partner, especially because a key component of this problem is that such persons become extremely anxious if sex is denied. They may present with multiple affairs or with constant demands on the partners. However, most people who have affairs do not have a sexual compulsion. Compulsive sexual behaviors over the Internet or compulsive viewing of pornography on the World Wide Web have become common presentations for sex therapy.

Treatment for sexual compulsions is still controversial. Some therapists use a Twelve-Step–based addiction model with group therapy; some treat it as a compulsion with individual therapy and medication (particularly selective serotonin reuptake inhibitors [SSRIs], such as fluoxetine). Couples therapy is still a critical component of treatment to educate the couple and, if multiple affairs have taken place, to discuss the viability of the marriage.

In recent years, emphasis has shifted to the role of biomedical and organic factors in the etiology of sexual dysfunction, along with the growing use of medical and surgical treatment interventions. Particular focus has been given to the role of vascular disorders and neuroendocrine problems, as well as the tendency for many medications to affect sexual functioning. It is critical for the patient to have a thorough physical workup. (For a good review on the interaction of medication and sexuality, see Abramowicz [1992].)

A variety of medical approaches to the treatment of erectile disorders in men have been developed in recent years. These include, but are not limited to, surgical prostheses and penile implants (seldom used in the last few years), intracorporal injection of vasoactive drugs such as papavarine, constriction rings and vacuum pump devices, and urethral suppositories. In 1998, oral medication for the treatment of impotence was introduced (sildenafil [Viagra]) and has become a useful tool in the treatment of male erectile difficulties. Surgical treatments are available for the correction of arterial insufficiency or venous leakage problems. These methods may be more or less acceptable both to the man and his partner. There has been some success in treating premature ejaculation with SSRIs and clomipramine; however, because these may also decrease sexual desire, caution and careful monitoring are indicated (Abramowicz 1992). Bupropion (Wellbutrin) is helpful in preventing loss of sexual desire or decrease of sexual functioning in patients treated with SSRIs (Rosen and Ashton 1993). Yohimbine is another helpful adjunct in some patients.

In women, most medical interventions have been for dyspareunia. Female dyspareunia due to decreased vaginal lubrication associated with declining of estrogen levels with age can be treated with topical estrogen cream or lubricant jelly. Even when an organic cause for dyspareunia is found and treated, the conditioned anxiety and lack of arousal associated with sex usually requires an additional course of couples therapy with a sexual focus. Hormone treatment for lack of desire has not proven effective (Rosen and Leiblum 1995), although it can be helpful in increasing vaginal lubrication.

■ OTHER ISSUES RELATED TO SEXUALITY AND MARRIAGE

Homosexuality and Bisexuality

Observations of human sexual behavior, affectional attachments, erotic fantasies, arousal, and erotic preference have suggested that sexual orientation and identity are not static. In fact, both may fluctuate over a person's lifetime. Sometimes changes in sexuality are only phases, whereas sometimes they become the predominant disposition of a person's sexual relations. Regardless, deviation from heterosexuality in Western society is frequently accompanied by rejection, not only by one's immediate family but also by one's peers and, in some cases, society in general. Bisexual persons may experience the additional lack of acceptance by gay and lesbian friends or associates, who may accuse them of fence-sitting, of sleeping with the enemy, or of being deviant because they are unable to choose to be heterosexual or homosexual. For the therapist, the issue should be centered on understanding and listening to the other's experiences even if they are quite different from his or her own.

Marital Issues in Homosexual or Bisexual Individuals

Many persons who are bisexual or whose homosexuality is admitted to consciousness later in life spend some years of their lives in heterosexual marriages. Many such persons are able to function well heterosexually, changing their sexual focus when they realize that something is missing or that their level of desire and love is greater for their own sex. Some have low levels of sexual desire in the marriage and develop affairs. Because there may be a great deal of love and affection between the marital partners, the discovery that one member is homosexual is very painful, and the desire to remain in the marriage may be strong on one or both sides. Although sex therapy can improve sexual functioning, there is no approach that has proved effective in decreasing homosexual desires and wishes. The couple must decide how to handle the situation—that is, to divorce, to remain in the relationship and allow for alternative sexual behaviors, or for the homosexual person to remain monogamous in the marriage and give up expressing the other parts of himself or herself. Therapy can help the couple clarify alternatives and make decisions. Unfortunately, even with the most loving spouses, the most common final event is divorce.

Sexual Functioning After Abuse and Rape

Rape and sexual abuse are acts of violence that have a serious impact on a person's ability to respond sexually in marriage. Both are likely to result in symptoms of posttraumatic stress disorder, producing anxiety and flashbacks when sex is initiated, even with a loved partner. Decreased sexual desire or sexual aversions are very common, although some women with a history of early sexual abuse become indiscriminately sexual, believing they are used merchandise and worthy only because of their sexuality.

Women with histories of early sexual abuse may have periods of relatively normal sexual functioning but may begin to have symptoms during therapy for other sequelae of the abuse (such as depression). This is because memories of the abuse are brought to the forefront of consciousness. In these cases, the husband must be carefully informed of what is happening so that he can have the patience to deal with his wife's varying moods and concerns. These symptoms usually change by the end of treatment.

For a previously well-functioning adult who has been raped, sexual symptoms may be either relatively brief or long-standing, depending on the circumstances of the rape, the amount of physical damage, the vulnerability of the victim, and the partner's response. Because the partners of rape victims also have a complex set of feelings, including a wish to protect, a sense of shame, and murderous rage toward the rapist, they may or may not be able to respond empathically as the victims deal with the trauma and their own feelings.

Couples therapy must be directed primarily toward helping the couple to respond to each other empathically and to deal with the meaning of the trauma. In some cases behavioral desensitization exercises may slow things down enough to make sex more comfortable.

Sexual Problems After Medical Illness

Adults treated for cancer, diabetes, heart disease, prostate disease, HIV, and chemical dependency may face special sexual challenges due to the underlying disorder, its treatment, or its effect on the couple's relationship. Two separate kinds of problems can occur. In one, the illness specifically affects sexual functioning. For example, surgery for prostate cancer may produce erectile dysfunction. This disorder is now generally treated medically with alprostadil or similar medication in various forms; in a few cases, penile prosthesis may be necessary. When a therapist is treating these patients, close communication with the urologist is necessary. The therapist should also help the partners to expand their repertoire of nonintercourse sexual behaviors. In the second type of problem, sex is still possible but the couple is anxious that having sex will injure the person. A classic example is sex after myocardial infarction (Cobb and Schaffer 1975). There is no evidence that sex with a known partner in familiar surroundings is problematic for the heart. The very few heart attacks related to sex are most likely to involve affair partners and heavy intake of food or alcohol. The couple should be advised to resume sex as soon as any reasonable exercise is permissible.

Likewise, erectile dysfunction may be the predictable side effect of certain antihypertensive medications. Narcotics such as heroin, barbiturates, and alcohol have a similar effect. Obviously, addictive drugs should be stopped or efforts made to change necessary medications. Many of the newer antidepressants can decrease sexual desire and delay orgasm. In general, the treatment of choice is to lower the dose or change antidepressants, although adjunctive pharmacologic therapy is sometimes helpful in reducing these side effects. Serious illness of any kind, in addition to treatment for certain illness such as cancer, may leave the person with no sexual interest. In this case, the couple may have to live with the situation, and the therapist's task is to help the couple to decide the best way to handle it within the marital relationship. Similarly, surgery, chemotherapy, or radiation for cervical, ovarian, or prostate cancer can reduce desire and performance. HIV and AIDS should alter a couple's approach to sex, and safe sexual practices must be recommended.

Sexual Problems in Elderly People

With the rapid growth in the number of elderly people, there has been an increased interest in their psychiatric and sexual problems.

Contrary to popular belief, however, sexual activity does not have to decrease once couples pass their forties. The family therapist can help couples realize the following:

- Advancing years are not a contraindication to sexuality and sensuality.
- It should be perfectly acceptable for the couple to have less frequent intercourse, but they should make efforts not to decrease their general level of affection.
- Older men may achieve erection and orgasm more slowly and may not necessarily ejaculate each time they have intercourse; older women may have a shorter excitement phase and their orgasms may be less intense and characterized by slower vaginal contractions. Both partners, however, can still have a regular, ongoing sexual life.

Even after an elderly patient has had a severe disability, such as a stroke, his or her sexual life can still be maintained. The couple can be aided in adjusting to changes of sexual functioning by thorough discussion of what positions and techniques are still possible.

■ REFERENCES

Abramowicz ME: Drugs that cause sexual dysfunction: an update. The Medical Letter: 34:95–111, 1992

American Psychiatric Association: Diagnostic and Statistical Manual of Mental Disorders, 4th Edition, Text Revision. Washington, DC, American Psychiatric Association, 2000, pp 535–582

Berman E, Hof H: The sexual genogram—assessing family of origin factors in the treatment of sexual dysfunction, in Integrating Sex and Marital Therapy: A Clinical Guide. Edited by Weeks G, Hof L. New York, Brunner/Mazel, 1987, pp 37–57

Cobb LA, Schaffer WE: Letter to the editor. New Engl J Med 293:1100, 1975

Kaplan HS: The Sexual Desire Disorders: Dysfunctional Regulation of Sexual Motivation. New York, Brunner/Mazel, 1995

Laumann EO, Gagnon JH, Michael RT, et al: The Social Organization of Sexuality: Sexual Practices in the United States. Chicago, IL, University of Chicago Press, 1994

Leiblum S, Rosen R: Principles and Practice of Sex Therapy, 2nd Edition. New York, Guilford, 1989

LoPiccolo J, Stock W: Treatment of sexual dysfunction. J Consult Clin Psychol 54:158–167, 1996

Masters W, Johnson V: Human Sexual Response. Boston, MA, Little, Brown, 1966

Rosen R, Ashton AK: Prosexual drugs: empirical status of the "new aphrodisiacs." Arch Sex Behav 22:521–543, 1993

Rosen R, Leiblum S: Treatment of sexual disorders in the 1990s: an integrated approach. J Consult Clin Psychol 63:877–890, 1995

Schnarch D: Passionate Marriage. New York, Norton, 1997

Zilbergeld B: The New Male Sexuality. New York, Bantam Books, 1992

13

SEPARATION AND DIVORCE

Separation and divorce are common occurrences in today's world. Many couples and families seek treatment during these phases of the relationship, since both separations and divorces cause stress for the couple, the children, and members of the extended family. The therapist must be ready to handle the many issues that develop as couples undergo these transitions.

■ SEPARATION

The process of separation may be an experiment on the part of a couple experiencing stress or the first step in a process leading directly to divorce. Trial separations in which the couple still expresses interest in rebuilding the marriage, and neither are having an affair, can be a chance for the therapist and couple to do serious work. In general, separations are to be avoided when possible, since the best therapy can usually be done when the couple is in constant contact. Separations may be unavoidable, or preferable, in situations of very high conflict, violence, or alcoholism, or when a person who married very young and feels as if he or she has no identity needs to be alone for a period of time. During a trial separation, the couple should be encouraged not to date others, to have ongoing couples therapy, and to have planned and scheduled times to be together during which they have some pleasant experiences as well as serious talks.

When a couple separates, the family therapist can help uncover the problems that prevent some people from living together successfully on a sustained basis. Maintaining a lasting relationship is often more difficult than forming a new one, and often both patients and therapists give up too quickly. Not everything can be changed, but some things can be improved, and the therapist must be realistic in helping the partners to accept the parts of themselves that cannot be changed. However, it is critical that the therapist not be the only one in the system trying to hold the relationship together. The decision of whether to separate must be made by the couple, not the therapist.

Couples who separate because one person has an active affair partner face a more difficult situation. The couple and the therapist must decide whether therapy is possible and whether ongoing contact between spouses is preferable. Separation and divorce also increase the risk of depression, more commonly in men than in women (Weissman et al. 1996).

■ SEPARATION LEADING TO DIVORCE

Once a couple has decided that divorce is inevitable, a different situation exists. The imminent dissolution of the family as it was (it has been said that every divorce is the death of a small civilization) produces violent feelings of abandonment, grief, and loss in family members, regardless of their age. Although it has been assumed that divorce is easier once late-teenage children have left home for college or work, even adults in their thirties are often deeply upset by their parents' divorce. The parents and siblings of each spouse may also have a variety of feelings, including anger and loss. Obviously, the partners initiating the divorce may have other feelings as well, such as relief, but loss is always present as well.

Of the various issues concerning divorce that are discussed, the most immediate have to do with finding separate living arrangements, dealing with children, and redistributing money. In general, men have less experience than women in dealing with issues concerning the children, and women have less experience and more fear around issues of money. If the husband has primarily left parenting to his wife, he must learn, and quickly, how to relate to his children when he is alone and must be actively encouraged to see them frequently and regularly and to be in contact with his wife about sharing the parenting responsibilities. Other issues that arise at this time are how long to live in the same house—in general, children should be given a few weeks to adjust to the situation rather than having the parent move out immediately after announcing the divorce. Remaining together for months once divorce has been chosen is often very destructive to both parties, although some couples in poor financial situations, or when both refuse to leave the home, have done this. The therapist must be very active during the early phases of separation to make sure that the children are cared for and not used as pawns. The therapist should also aid the couple in making coherent, not emotionally driven, decisions in areas such as the redistribution of money. It is usually best to postpone any major decisions, such as selling the house or giving up one's job, until the dust settles. In some cases, legal advice about customary legal arrangements in the patient's location should be sought even if divorce has not been initiated.

Once a couple has decided to divorce, they often drop out of therapy. They should be encouraged to remain in treatment at least long enough to plan their initial moves concerning telling the children and their families of origin, to make initial financial arrangements, and to discuss how to handle the physical separation. Some couples may want to review the course of the marriage to further understand what went wrong, but for most couples emotions are too high at this time. Either or both partners may request individual therapy; sometimes a support group for separating and divorcing people is also helpful. If the couple has been seen conjointly, in some situations it is helpful to refer them to different therapists rather than have the former couple's therapist do the individual work. In other cases, the couple's therapist may continue with one member (or, rarely, both). If only one person is seen by the original couple's therapist, the other may feel that it is unfair, but some spouses are relieved when their former mate continues in therapy. It is almost impossible to see both members of a divorcing couple individually, because the therapist is now privy to information about legal and custody battles from both sides. In addition, the spouses may see their former couple's therapist as a link to or as favoring the other and thus may not be able to fully engage in their own work.

Communicating the Issue of Divorce to Children

Telling the children is usually a traumatic event for the parents. It is useful to remember that, like many other issues, this is a process and not a single event. Initially, most children hear very little aside from the fact that divorce is impending. Children do not really know what it will mean for them until they have lived with it, and usually do not know what questions to ask at first. This must be discussed again and again in the ensuing weeks, as plans are made. The information that must be conveyed, either all at once or over time, includes the following:

- We are getting a divorce. That means we won't be living together.
- We will always be your parents, and we both love you. That does not change.
- You will not have to choose between us. [This may or may not be true, and the therapist must help the couple keep the children out of the middle.]
- You did not cause this divorce and could not have prevented it.
- As time goes on, we will need to keep talking about what is happening with all of us, both the feelings and the changes in our lives. We will talk about what is happening with us, and you need to talk about what you need. You can also talk to your friends and whoever else it would help to talk to.

The children need to be told, as simply as possible and in an age-appropriate fashion, the reasons for the divorce. Teenage children in particular want a reasonable amount of information. If any parent is having an active affair, it is not unusual for one or more of the children to be aware of it. Children tend to overhear conversations and to know what is going on with their parents to a larger extent than parents are aware. Trying to keep secret the major reasons for the divorce is impossible. Because children today usually have friends whose parents are divorced, there are fewer stigmas and more knowledge than a generation or two ago. On the other hand, no child wants the details of their parents' sexual or intimate lives. Children need to be reminded that at the time of their birth, their parents loved one another and that the children were wanted; communicating this can help to alleviate children's fear that they were in some way responsible for the divorce.

Children are, appropriately, also concerned about the details of their daily lives—who will care for them and pick them up at school, where they will keep their pets, and whether they will have to leave their house. For most children, the house and neighborhood are a crucial part of their sense of self. They need to be reassured that, whatever the living arrangements, they will be considered and taken care of.

Generally, it is best for both parents to be present when the initial announcement is made to the children so that everyone hears the same information. However, private talks later are also necessary and appropriate, because each parent must now learn how to parent alone. Parents need to check with each other before conveying potentially explosive information about financial changes or about an affair partner.

Immediate Issues

The level of conflict during the initial year of living apart varies greatly depending on whether the divorce is sudden or has been long in the planning, whether one spouse opposes it, and what the level of preseparation conflict was like. Regardless of whether the divorce was planned for, the many changes in feelings and life structure make the situation difficult. If the couple has a fair amount of goodwill left, or if one partner is so guilty that he or she agrees to almost anything, many decisions can be made quickly. Most often, each decision is complex and will be struggled over.

In general, the early months of the separation are likely to cause irrational behavior between the ex-partners, regardless of how well each person is managing children or work. For many people, the first months in particular are a crazy time, when everything feels upside down. The job of the therapist is to keep each person grounded, allowing him or her to tell the story over and over and to find answers to the questions "How did this happen?" and "Am I still a good person?"

For the couple, mediation is often helpful in problem solving. The more the couple can make decisions themselves with a mediator's help, rather than using the judicial system, the better. If mediation does not work, however, supporting the process of finding and working with a lawyer may be helpful. For many, this is a first-time experience with the legal process. The ex-partners may be overwhelmed and unable to be an advocate for their own interests with the lawyer.

Family conflict may escalate during the year after divorce, although for high-conflict families it may decrease. If the parents are having a difficult time, they may temporarily find that their parental skills decrease and may become inconsistent, less affectionate, and less focused on discipline and continuity. Parental quarreling and mutual denigration can lead to children becoming anxious, feeling that they must take sides, or in the case of latency and early adolescent children, completely cutting off the absent parent. Statistically, the risk of delinquency is greater when the parents separate or divorce than when a parent dies. The parameters of marital discord that seem most toxic for children are prolonged marital disputes, parental pathology that impinges on the child's functioning, and lack of a good relationship with either parent. Rapid changes in lifestyle and finances are stressful for everyone and add to frustration. However, the situation may improve in many families, particularly those in which the parent who is leaving has been violent, alcoholic, or emotionally abusive. Fathers who have left the active parenting to their wives may improve their parenting when they have the children by themselves. Many families, after an initial period of disruption, do very well.

Therapy for Families Facing Divorce

Common treatment alternatives for the family facing divorce may include 1) no formal treatment, 2) couple work with discussion about the children, 3) family treatment with both ex-spouses and the children, or 4) work with the children and only one parent on issues that each parent has with the children. Family therapy must have a carefully composed agenda that is focused primarily on practical issues, such as living arrangements, handling transfers of children between parents, emergencies, and discipline. Central issues are what the children need and whether they are caught between the parents—for instance, whether they have been asked to "tattle" on a parent or to ask one parent for money for the other. Therapy must be clearly focused on the children's problems and not on rehashing the marriage. Although the same therapist can see each parent alone with the children, he or she must also have knowledge and respect for the other partner. The therapist is likely to worsen the struggles between the spouses if he or she begins working with the custodial parent and children after a divorce and does not speak to or meet with the noncustodial parent or consider that person's concerns. *The Difficult Divorce*, by Isaacs et al. (1986), is a good reference for therapists working with couples with no ability to compromise or deal with each other. For the children alone, intervention is also possible but not mandatory. It may include a children's support group or individual therapy. It is also important to inform others who have contact with the child, especially the school, that this event has occurred in the child's life.

One very difficult issue is that of introducing the child to new love relationships for one or both parents. Children may not want to meet the new lover of a parent, particularly if this person was an affair partner for whom the parent left the marriage. Even if children are ready, the ex-spouse may be furious about having the children meet the affair partner, whom he or she may see as immoral or evil. However, if the children are to have a relationship with both parents, they must eventually find some way to deal with the new lover, at least with regard if not affection. The therapist must help the family to deal with the realities of the situation, although it is generally wise to wait at least a few months after a separation before introducing the new person if there is a great deal of animosity. New relationships should not be introduced to the children unless they are potentially serious ones. If possible, live-in status should be reserved for new partners who are clear that they intend to marry—otherwise, their ambiguous status in the house may lead to real problems with the children. Sleepover status is a highly emotional topic, and no clear guidelines are obvious in most situations—a good rule of thumb is not to have a new partner stay overnight unless the relationship has reached a relatively committed status.

■ DIVORCE, SINGLE-PARENT AND BINUCLEAR FAMILIES, STEPFAMILIES, AND COHABITING COUPLES

The fact of divorce should not lead one to think only of pathological sequelae, because a conflict-ridden, intact family can be more detrimental to a child than is a stable home in which the parents are divorced. As such, divorce can be a positive solution to a destructive family situation. This seems to be especially true in the presence of a rejecting, demeaning, or psychiatrically ill parent.

Very little is known about the very-long-term phase of the divorce process. No studies have been carried out in which divorced parents are compared with discordant parents who contemplate divorce but stay together, or with discordant parents who have never considered divorce. The work of Wallerstein (1988) suggests that some children of divorced families have strong feelings about it even 10 years later. That author conducted a systematic follow-up of a small sample of children of divorce (with no control subjects) and found that 1) three in five children felt rejected by at least one of the parents, 2) in at least half the families both parents remained angry, and 3) depending on age, as expected, children conceptualize and feel differently about divorce. Wallerstein (1988) suggested that divorcing parents apologize for the pain they are causing their children, express their own sadness to allow children to express their feelings about the ending of the relationship, and give children concrete details about future plans as soon as possible. Her age-specific comments include the following:

- *Adolescent.* Try not to lean on the child for support—don't get lost in your own needs to the detriment of helping the adolescent deal with his or her own needs.
- *Ages 9–12.* The angriest children tend to take sides and to act as though they understand the issue when they may actually understand very little. These children need to be told not to get involved in the parents' fight.
- *Younger children.* Reassure the children that they will still have both a mother and a father. At this age, abandonment can be a central issue. For the preschooler, continued ongoing contact from both parents on a regular and frequent basis is best.

It must be kept in mind that the above comments are generalizations. For example, although abandonment is preeminent in younger children, it is not uncommon for older children and adolescents to experience similar feelings. In addition, family stressors often cause children to regress, emotionally as well as behaviorally, to earlier stages of development.

Single-Parent and Binuclear Families

Although the general rules of family treatment apply to all families, single-parent and binuclear families[1] that have been formed subsequent to divorce are subject to certain kinds of additional stress. Single-parent families must be carefully evaluated to determine who is in

---

[1]*Binuclear family* refers to a divorced family in which both parents remain central in the children's lives. One or both parents may remarry; the binuclear family would then expand to include a stepparent and possibly stepsiblings or half siblings.

the functioning system. A parent with legal custody of children may be living with his or her parent, a lover, or a friend. Even if the non-custodial parent visits infrequently, he (usually it is a male) may still be very important in the child's life. Alternatively, the single parent and the children may form a tightly self-contained unit.

Hierarchy is a complex issue in single-parent families. A grandparent may take over a major portion of the childrearing duties, especially if the parent and children are living in the grandparent's house. A lover may feel that he or she should take over disciplinary duties without any clear mandate to do so. Because the custodial parent may be overwhelmed by a combination of work and household duties, it is not uncommon for one or more of the children to act as companion to the parent or as surrogate parent to younger children. In other cases, the family may operate with a high level of democracy in which all children share more of the power and responsibility than in a two-adult household. However, if conflicts occur, it should be clear that the custodial parent has the final say in the matter. Children must not be overburdened with parenting responsibilities. Yet children are capable of taking on a reasonable share of the chores when it is obvious that help is needed. For many children, a single-parent family is one in which their contribution is needed and welcomed.

In therapy, it is important to speak to all family members rather than only to a parent or one child. If the family is living with grandparents, it is important to include the grandparent(s) in at least some of the meetings. The therapist must be willing to work with the family to determine the best system available, rather than assuming the parent must carry the entire burden himself or herself.

If the parent, particularly a single mother, has no supports, she is prone to depression and demoralization. The therapist's job is to help her to form a functioning support system rather than to try to be the support system themselves.

In binuclear families, the central issues involve the multiple systems in which the children must operate. Not only must the parents collaborate on clear rules for the children, but if one or both remarry, the new spouses will also be involved. Examples of goals for remarried couples are presented in Table 13–1.

TABLE 13–1. **Therapy goals for remarried couples**

1. To consolidate the remarried couple as a unit and their authority in the system, helping the two adults to understand and develop a modus operandi to further their romantic love requirements and their necessity to parent.

2. To consolidate the parental authority in the system among biological parents and stepparents with the formation of a collaborative coparenting team.

3. As a corollary to item 2, to help children deal with and minimize the continuance and exacerbation of loyalty binds between their two biological parents and between the biological parent and the ipsilateral stepparent.

4. To facilitate mourning of the nuclear family, former partner, old neighborhoods, friends, and way of life. A period of mourning prepares the way to accept and to grow with the new reality of remarriage.

5. To ensure that there is a secure place for the child's development and to maximize the potential within both family systems. It is hoped that the two systems can be synergistic at the same time the child learns that there is not just one way of dealing with many life situations.

6. To accept and integrate the child's need for individuation from both families and for more peer involvement. A corollary to this is the child who prematurely develops great peer involvement when it was not possible to find appropriate love and nurturance in the household system of either biological parent. One approach may be to strengthen the bond and acceptance of the child in one if not both family systems.

7. To help family members accept and tolerate their differences from some idealized nuclear family model

---

In single-parent families, the launching of children, particularly the oldest, is often problematic because they have been such crucial supports for the parent and younger children. Often, the oldest child becomes symptomatic just before he or she is ready to leave for college, as a way of testing whether it is safe to go.

Stepfamilies

Because of their different structure, stepfamilies need to be evaluated and treated within the context of awareness of appropriate stepfamily norms. Using a nuclear family model can lead stepfamily members to pursue unrealistic goals, with unfortunate consequences.

The complexities and intricacies of stepfamily relationships appear to require a systemic perspective, even when the therapist is working with a single individual from a stepfamily "suprasystem" (Sager et al. 1983). The therapist must think in terms of the family, regardless of who or how many are being seen. This approach is also important when the stepfamily has multiple problems. In addition to other types of interventions (e.g., for drug abuse or chronic illness), dealing with stepfamily dynamics and issues can reduce tensions, thus giving family members more energy to deal with their other difficulties.

The question of whom to see in therapy is important. It can be detrimental to see the new couple and the children together in the same session before the couple has arrived at the stage of family integration in which they have some ability to be supportive of one another and to work together on family issues. Seeing the couple alone is an important way to demonstrate the importance of the couple and to help the two individuals to strengthen their relationship. Some therapists meet with all members of the *metafamily*—that is, all those who are involved with the children, such as ex-spouses, lovers, and stepparents.

Even when a couple is working well together, stepfamily relationships do not necessarily develop spontaneously. The family may need inclusive family therapy to work out these relationships. Communication and special one-to-one time between parents and children, and between stepparents and stepchildren, can be important in building and maintaining relationships. For children in stepfamilies, this can reduce the loss of previously more exclusive parental attention and can foster communication and bonding between stepparents and stepchildren.

The balance of power does not initially reside with the couple in stepfamilies. Stepparents join children with a parent who, as far as the children are concerned, has no authority. Many remarried parents make the error of expecting the stepparent to take on a disciplinary role with the children. Research indicates that a stepparent needs to come in slowly before becoming a comanager with the biological parent, who needs to become, or remain, the active parenting adult with his or her children and also needs to require civil behavior in the household. These steps can create a climate in which stepfamily relationships can develop and the stepparent can begin to take on a comanagement role with the biological parent. With young children, this process may take 1–2 years (Stern 1978); with older children, it usually takes longer (Papernow 1993).

A great deal of the complexity in remarried families stems from the fact that there are more than two parenting adults in the children's lives. With a biological parent in another household, there may be three or four parenting adults if both parents are remarried, and children may be living part of the time in each of these two households. When parents feel insecure, they tend to fear the loss of their children's love to the other parent and perhaps to that parent's new partner. Another concern is the loss of control and sense of helplessness that arises because of the mere existence of the other household. In this case the therapeutic task is to help the couple to build an adequate boundary around its household and to learn to respect that of the other household. In addition, gates in the boundaries are needed for the children so they can come and go comfortably. Adults often need help in controlling the things that they can control in their own home and letting go of concerns about situations in the other household. Gaining control and accepting the limits of their influence is helpful in reducing their feelings of helplessness.

Forming a parenting coalition of parents and stepparents can be difficult, but with help it is possible (Visher and Visher 1988, 1990). Ordinarily this requires the new couple to develop a solid, secure bond before they are emotionally able to form a working relationship with the children's other household. The less the hostility between their households, the fewer the loyalty conflicts on the part of the children and the more satisfaction of all the adults. In some situations it can be helpful to bring all the adults together to work on issues involving the children. Bringing them together in therapy becomes a possibility when the partners in each couple have formed a strong bond with each other. The therapist needs to make direct, personal contact with each household, state clearly the purpose of the joint meeting, and then make certain that the agenda of the session does not include potentially explosive areas that are unconnected with the present welfare of the child. Older children may need to be included when their situations are being discussed.

The emotional climate in stepfamilies is often intense, particularly during the early stages of stepfamily integration. A helpful way to conceptualize the reasons for this intensity is to understand and recognize the inability of new stepfamilies to meet three very basic human emotional needs:

1. To belong to a group
2. To be cared about and loved by a few special people
3. To have some control over one's life

Because of all the changes and unfamiliarity in the household, stepfamily members can feel out of control, not accepted by the new people in their lives, and as though they do not belong in this unfamiliar group. Many parents who have remarried fear the loss of their children, whom they love and by whom they are loved. Stepparents in particular feel unloved, alienated from the group, and with little control. Children are upset by their lack of control over all the losses and events occurring in their lives.

For therapists, then, the basic task is to help the family members to gain an understanding of these basic emotional needs so that they can have empathy for everyone else in the family and can be understood in return. The family needs to find ways in which to communicate, fill in past history with one another, and further accelerate the sense of control and belonging by developing rituals and predictable day-to-day ways of doing things. Being cared about requires the building of relationships. This takes time and positive shared memories, both on a one-to-one basis and as a family unit.

Many stepfamilies who come for therapy need the therapist to validate their feelings and the worth and viability of their family, to normalize the situations that arise in such families, to find ways to deal effectively with the challenges, and to find support for the new couple relationship. With this assistance, remarried families can work toward satisfactory integration, deal more effectively with disruptive situations, and bring satisfaction and happiness to the adults and the children.

Cohabiting Couples

Cohabitation, once seen as pathology, sin, or nonconformity, is now a common developmental phase for young people developing intimacy or older people after divorce. Our estimate is that about 50% of marrying couples have lived together for some time before marriage. Cohabiting couples that come for therapy are most likely to present with the need to determine the future of the relationship. Couples who have been living together for some time and are unable to make the decision to marry tend to be divided into those with one committed and one uncommitted partner and those in which both partners have felt the relationship to be unsatisfactory but are afraid to be on their own. Therapy consists of clarifying each partner's position and helping the couple think through what would have to occur in order to make the relationship go forward (or to end).

■ REFERENCES

Isaacs M, Montalvo B, Abelsohn D: The Difficult Divorce: Therapy for Children and Families. New York, Basic Books, 1986

Papernow P: Becoming a Stepfamily: Patterns of Development in Remarried Families. San Francisco, CA, Jossey-Bass, 1993

Sager CJ, Brown HS, Crohn H, et al: Treating the Remarried Family. New York, Brunner/Mazel, 1983

Stern PA: Stepfather families: integration around child discipline. Issues Ment Health Nurs 1:50–56, 1978

Visher EB, Visher JS: Old Loyalties, New Ties: Therapeutic Strategies With Stepfamilies. New York, Brunner/Mazel, 1988

Visher EB, Visher JS: Parenting coalitions after remarriage: dynamics and therapeutic guidelines. Fam Relat 38:65–70, 1990

Wallerstein J: Second Chances. New York, Ticknor and Fields, 1988

Weissman MM, Bland RC, Canino GJ, et al: Cross-national epidemiology of major depression and bipolar disorder. JAMA 276:293–299, 1996

INDICATIONS AND CONTRAINDICATIONS FOR FAMILY THERAPY

Although we believe strongly that couples or family therapy is indicated for most marital and family problems and should be included at some point in the treatment of many psychiatric conditions (including major Axis I disorders such as schizophrenia), there are still many questions in the field. For persons with significant personal issues as well as family issues, what is the relationship among individual therapy, family therapy, group therapy, and medication? If other treatment modalities are indicated, how does one decide whether to use them concurrently or consecutively?

■ MARITAL THERAPY

Marital Conflict and Dissatisfaction

There is one area in which a growing body of research has produced consistent results—the treatment of marital difficulties. For many years it has been a prevalent clinical opinion that marital therapy is the treatment of choice for marital difficulties. Other treatment modalities may be used simultaneously or sequentially.

> A couple came in seeking treatment because of a sense of distance and sadness in their relationship. History revealed that the husband was suffering depression precipitated by the death of his father

2 years before. His relationship with his father had been very poor and was unresolved at the time of the father's death.

Possible treatment plans in this case include the following:

- Couples work, which includes an in-depth discussion of both partners' early history and the husband's grief and loss during the course of the couple's therapy. Medication might be included in this plan if indicated.
- Concurrent individual and couples work.
- Individual work with the husband first, perhaps including medication, dealing with issues around his father, followed by couples therapy if still indicated.
- Family-of-origin therapy with the husband and his mother and sibling in order to do grief work and help resolve remaining family issues.

Guidelines in this case include the following:

1. Make the decision with the couple's participation.
2. Do the most urgent thing first.

In this case the couple felt that, unless the marriage was attended to, it was rapidly headed for divorce. The therapist chose to begin with couples therapy, focusing on ways in which the husband could share his feelings with his wife, how he could be there for her despite his sadness, and his wife's grief and anger at having a depressed husband, given her own history of growing up with a depressed father. They then began to discuss both families of origin. The wife, who knew the husband's family conflict well, was able to offer a number of suggestions about the origin of the problem and how grieving might begin. The therapist later saw the husband alone for several sessions and had two family-of-origin sessions with the husband, his mother, and his brother.

More complex situations occur when the couple is in serious conflict over goals. This is most difficult when one partner wants to preserve the marriage and the other is very ambivalent but probably wants to divorce. In this case, the therapist must determine whether it is best to see the ambivalent person alone to sort out his or her feelings or whether to work on the marital relationship directly and deal with ambivalence within the couples work.

Sexual Issues

Sexual issues are almost always dealt with conjointly if possible, and research suggests that therapy must be directed to both couple dynamics and sexual symptoms. However, therapy does not have to include sensate focus exercises unless indicated for specific problems. Again, however, some people need time alone to consider their previous sexual experiences, fantasies, and feelings.

Families in the Process of Divorce

Families in the process of divorce require a complicated mix of individual and family work. Although the grief work involving a separation is best done alone, attention to the details of establishing child care, new routines, and a way to communicate require joint work. It is critical that all those who are involved in child care have an opportunity to plan so that they do not lose the sense of the entire family's needs and positions.

In couples considering but not yet at the point of divorce, the issues of the couple versus those of the individual are complex. As stated previously, we know that individual therapy, which promotes personal growth in one partner without including or even informing the other, is more likely than couples therapy to lead to a split. Equally important, if individual therapy is indicated, the other partner (and the partner's therapist, if there is one) should be brought into the information loop.

■ THE CHILD AS THE IDENTIFIED PATIENT

When a child is the identified patient, it has long been the practice of child guidance clinics to involve at least one of the parents, usually in collateral treatment in which the patient and the parent both receive individual treatment but with different therapists. A more thoroughgoing approach, however, seems indicated in these cases, including an evaluation of the possible role of the child as the symptom bearer of more general family problems (often unresolved marital issues). Usually the marital partners are seen as a couple for a major part of the treatment. The child may benefit from some individual attention addressed to his or her particular symptoms and psychosocial difficulties. A common sequence of events is for the entire family to start out in treatment together, and then for various individual dyads and triads to be separated out for special attention after an interval of time. Of these, the marital dyad is unquestionably the most important. Some family therapists suggest that whenever there is a symptomatic child who is prepubescent, family treatment is indicated unless there are specific contraindications.

■ THE ADOLESCENT AS THE IDENTIFIED PATIENT

With the adolescent as the identified patient, focus on the family is still indicated, especially while the adolescent is living at home and has not yet established psychosocial autonomy. A good deal of attention must often be focused on the marital partnership. The adolescent often benefits from individual attention, as well as from the encouragement of peer group relationships.

There seems to be some growing consensus that family therapy is most indicated when the symptomatic adolescent is exhibiting acting-out behavior. Some adolescents are seen who are unequipped to deal with symbolic psychological processes and are not able to benefit from insight-oriented individual modes of treatment. A more focused, action-oriented family model is often more helpful.

■ OTHER INTIMATE INTERPERSONAL SYSTEMS

Other systems that have at times been the focus of couple and family therapy include unmarried couples, and parents and their adult children.

Couples

Unmarried couples presenting for therapy for commitment and communication problems are treated, as are any couples. More complex situations emerge when one member of the couple is still married to someone else, or when the relationship is extremely inappropriate or in its very early stages.

Family-of-Origin Issues

The idea of seeing adult children with their parents is little known outside the family field. Adults are presumed to be able to report correctly about their childhood, and parents who have unfinished business with their children are expected to work on their own issues. However, whatever the dynamics of childhood, the real relationship of adult children and their parents is very meaningful and is best worked on by the people involved. This is particularly true because the parent, as well as the child, may have greatly changed in the 20 or 30 years since the child has grown. Although we do not have quantitative research on this issue, we do have years of clinical experience strongly suggesting that family sessions, if respectful and supportive, can powerfully turn around many highly dysfunctional family dynamics and allow parents and children to make some kind of peace with each other. In addition, the process of learning about one's past from one's parents and seeing them as the flawed but real people they are and were, rather than the monsters of one's childhood, often speeds the process of one's own therapy.

■ SITUATIONS IN WHICH FAMILY THERAPY IS DIFFICULT AND PERHAPS CONTRAINDICATED

Psychopathology in One Family Member Makes Family Therapy Ineffective

Dishonesty or manipulation of the therapy for secondary gain would constitute a serious handicap to effective treatment. For example, a partner might use therapy as a way to keep a spouse involved while continuing to conceal an affair. Some persons, such as those with antisocial personality disorders, are good at convincing others of the honesty of their position while engaging in very destructive behavior (e.g., using the family's money to gamble or engaging in crime). Children who are lying or stealing, however, are most likely responding to family issues, and these family issues must be addressed in therapy.

If one family member is extremely paranoid, manic, or agitated, medication should be initiated before the onset of family therapy for behavior that is too disruptive to control. However, as pointed out in an earlier chapter, even quite psychotic people can be active members of the family and can profit from family work.

There is still controversy over the role of family therapy for substance-abusing persons (Stanton 1995). In some cases, particularly when the user is an adolescent or a young adult and is not physically dependent on the drug, family therapy may be a primary modality of treatment. For more severely addicted people, family therapy must be part of a larger treatment plan including detoxification, group, and specific alcohol and drug treatment.

Family or Therapist Believes the Risks of Therapy Would Outweigh the Advantages

Family members may be concerned that treatment will leave them in a worse state than when they began. These possibilities should be explored at the outset, and when possible, the therapist should be very sensitive to these concerns. This concern is very common when families apply to a child guidance clinic. Many children develop problems in relation to parental conflicts. For example, a child may become school phobic, abusive to other children, or encopretic whenever the parents have severe fights. The parents may want the child "fixed" but may be determined not to address their conflicts because they are afraid that doing so will end in divorce. This is particularly true if the parents believe that one of them would become suicidal or psychotic if problems were admitted. In these cases, the therapy should be addressed only to parenting issues, and couple issues should be tabled, at least until the child is better. It is possible in most cases to find some way of uniting the parents around the child even when they are still in conflict.

> A 10-year-old girl whose problems included severe tantrums at home described her evenings. She would be doing her homework in the kitchen and her parents would have screaming fights in the next room, threatening each other with divorce. Needless to say, not much homework got done. She would often try to stop the fights, and sometimes the parents would appeal to her to settle the arguments. The parents admitted that they "fought" but downplayed the significance or level of verbal violence. The therapist framed the child as "sensitive" and asked the child to go to her room upstairs and close the door if her parents started to disagree. Her parents were asked to reward her when she did this so that she would not feel she was deserting them. Because they wanted her to do her homework more than they wanted a referee, they complied. Although the child's home life remained difficult, this at least got her out of the middle of things and allowed her some safe time, and she calmed down considerably. The parents' concerns could now be addressed to the extent that they were willing to do so. They chose to end therapy shortly thereafter.

A family that truly believes that therapy will result in divorce will not enter treatment. For couples and families in pain, the real issue is how hard and when to push the issues that they are afraid to discuss. For example, encouraging a woman who has been subservient to stand up for herself may provoke serious reprisals from a husband who needs a very acquiescent wife. As described in Chapter 15, this is both an ethical decision and a therapeutic one. In this case, as in others, it is best to discuss with the couple the pros and cons of changes in the relationship. Often the couple elects to stop therapy at the time and return to treatment later when the situation has deteriorated to the point that change is inevitable.

■ SKILLS AND ATTRIBUTES OF THE THERAPIST AS THEY AFFECT FAMILY WORK

Many therapists are uncomfortable with family groups or with particular types of families and should not force themselves to treat them. Therapists must be aware of family issues and refer patients for family therapy when needed.

> Mr. Q, age 35 years, was in individual treatment for 6 years for his depression. His therapist believed that he was passive and encouraged him to learn to speak up for what he wanted. Mr. Q and his wife went to couples therapy with an unrelated therapist at a point at which his wife was ready to leave the marriage. Mrs. Q said that her husband had always been self-centered, but in the years since therapy started he had been impossibly critical and demanding.
>
> In the couple's session, far from being passive, Mr. Q was angry, condescending, and completely unempathic to his wife. The individual therapist's disinterest in Mr. Q's perception of the problem had led to an increasingly dysfunctional marriage and near-divorce.

A decision to treat an individual should not mean ignoring couples issues. If a therapist has strong emotional ties to a family (e.g., a spouse, friend, or relative) or significant countertransference to a particular family, he or she should refer the family.

The age, sex, and race of the therapist can have significant effects on treatment, and these issues need to be considered. For example, a 50-year-old educated and status-conscious couple is not likely to respond to a 25-year-old therapist who has an M.S.W. rather than a Ph.D. degree. Many families of color, having experienced serious oppression, are reluctant to allow a middle-class white therapist to treat them without a long period of trust building.

■ CLINICAL IMPLICATIONS OF DATA FROM FAMILY THERAPY OUTCOME STUDIES

Pinsof and Wynne (1995) provide an overview of another perspective focused on the research data for the family therapist. We present the following important implications for family therapists (Pinsof and Wynne 1995, pp. 603–605):

> The following conclusions are based on an overview of the field of [marital and family therapy (MFT)] research. These conclusions are provisional; the field of MFT research is not ready for definitive conclusions at this stage of its development. Even though a considerable body of empirical evidence has been accumulated, most of the findings have not been replicated systematically. Additionally, even though the field has made great progress, many methodological problems still plague the research and hinder the accumulation of a coherent and clear body of knowledge about the efficacy and effectiveness of MFT. A strong conclusion requires confirmation from at least two controlled studies.
>
> 1. MFT works. A clear and consistent body of evidence has been accumulated and reviewed that indicates that MFT [marital therapy (MT)/family therapy (FT)] is significantly and clinically more efficacious than no psychotherapy for the following patients, disorders, and problems: adults schizophrenia (FT); outpatient depressed women in distressed marriages (MT); marital distress and conflict (MT): adult alcoholism and drug abuse (FT/MT); adult hypertension (MT); elderly dementia (FT); anorexia in young adolescent girls (FT); adolescent drug abuse (FT); child conduct disorders (FT); aggression and noncompliance in [attention deficit/hyperactivity disorder (ADHD)] children (FT); childhood autism (FT); chronic physical illnesses in children (asthma, diabetes, etc.) (FT); child obesity (FT); and cardiovascular risk factors in children (FT).
> 2. MFT is not harmful. MFT does not appear to have negative or destructive effects. In all of the research reviewed, there has not been one replicated and controlled study in which patients and families receiving family or marital therapy had poorer outcomes than patients receiving no therapy.
> 3. MFT is more efficacious than standard and/or individual treatments for the following patients, disorders, and problems: adult schizophrenia; depressed outpatient

women in distressed marriages; marital distress; adult alcoholism and drug abuse; adolescent conduct disorders; adolescent drug abuse; anorexia in young adolescent females; childhood autism; and various chronic physical illnesses in adults and children. Additionally, involving the family in engaging alcoholic adults in treatment is more efficacious than just working with the individual adults. Similarly, family involvement in aftercare for alcoholic adults is more efficacious than standard individual or group aftercare.

4. There are no scientific data at this time to support the superiority of any particular form of marital or family therapy over any other. The meta-analyses of MFT, when controlled from methodological confounds, failed to reveal any consistent effects of one type of MFT over another. Similarly, specific reviews did not reveal any consistent effects of one MFT approach over any other. The one trend and very preliminary hypothesis that emerged fairly consistently is that treatments that combined conventional family or marital therapy sessions with other interventions were more efficacious than standard family therapy approaches alone for severe disorders. It is premature to draw firm conclusions from this trend since it has not been formally tested in replicated controlled trials.

5. Data from a small number of studies indicate that MFT is more cost effective than standard inpatient and/or residential treatment/placement for schizophrenia and severe adolescent conduct disorders and delinquency. There are some preliminary data that suggest it is more cost effective than alternative treatments for adult alcoholism and adult and adolescent drug abuse. From the perspective of the health care providers and managed care, marital and family therapies may be more cost effective than individual treatments in that more clients or patients are treated by a therapist in a single session. Additionally, the broader systemic focus of many marital and family therapies means that the therapist is focused not only on the mental and physical health of the individual client but

also on the health of the other family members. This broader scope of concern theoretically expands the impact of MFT.

6. Marital and family therapy are not sufficient in itself to treat effectively a variety of severe disorders and problems. More than half of the treatments that have demonstrated efficacy involve components that go beyond the standard and conventional family therapy session format of MFT. All of the asterisked problems and disorders in this volume involve treatments that do more than just family therapy. For instance, in addition to the family therapy component, psychoeducational therapies for schizophrenia involve medication and educational components. Similarly, the most effective treatments for childhood autism, severe adolescent conduct disorders, adult and adolescent drug abuse, and adult alcoholism involve additional treatment (group and/or individual and/or medication) and education components.

The research on these problems and treatments suggests that family involvement is a critical and necessary component in the treatment of these problems but is not sufficient in itself. An emerging hypothesis from these data is that multi-component, integrative, and problem-focused treatments may be necessary to treat severe behavioral disorders effectively in adults, adolescents, and children. In fact, the more severe, pervasive, and disruptive the disorder, the greater the need to include multiple components in effective treatments.

■ REFERENCES

Pinsof WM, Wynne LC: The efficacy of marital and family therapy: an empirical review, conclusions and recommendations. J Marital Fam Ther 21:585–613, 1995

Stanton MD: Family therapy for drug abuse. Paper presented at the National Conference on Marital and Family Therapy Outcome and Process Research: State of the Science, Philadelphia, PA, 1995

ETHICAL AND PROFESSIONAL ISSUES IN FAMILY THERAPY

■ ETHICAL ISSUES INHERENT IN FAMILY THERAPY

The fundamental ethical dilemmas inherent in psychotherapy—confidentiality, limits of control, duty to warn and reporting of abuse, and therapist-patient boundaries—become more complex when the treatment involves more than one person. The family therapist has an ethical responsibility to everyone in the family. In some cases, individual needs and family system needs may be in conflict. For example, a husband may wish to conceal a brief episode of unprotected sex with another woman, whereas his wife is better protected, for health reasons as well as psychological reasons, if she knows about it. A wife's wish to be divorced from a psychiatrically ill and demanding husband may conflict with his need for her care. Such clinical situations provide a set of ethical dilemmas for the therapist.

The therapist must be clear that his or her job in most cases (such as impending divorce) is to help the partners sort out their values, obligations, and options rather than to make a decision for them. In some cases, however (such as the reporting of child abuse), the ethical decision must be the therapist's. In other instances, the therapist faces difficult gray areas in which decisions must be made on a case-by-case basis. The therapist also has certain unalterable ethical obligations, such as not engaging in dual relationships (see section on dual relationships later in this chapter) with patients or exploiting them for the therapist's own benefit. Although the operative concept is "first do no harm," the issues of how one defines harm, and who will or will not be harmed by a certain action, are complex and difficult questions.

Conflicting Interests of Family Members

It is not unusual for the interests of various family members to conflict at some point. Boszormenyi-Nagy and Spark (1973) emphasized years ago the contractual obligations and accountability between persons in the multiple generations of a family. The family therapist in this view is uniquely attuned to the well-being of all the family members (who will be affected by the treatment process) via their deep-rooted relatedness over time and through many generations. Relational ethics is concerned with the balance of equitable fairness between people. To gauge the balance of fairness in the here and now and across time and generations, each family member must consider both his or her own interests and the interests of each of the other family members. The basic issue is one of equitability—that is, everyone is entitled to have his or her welfare and interests considered in a way that is fair to the related interests of the other family members.

As we have discussed in previous chapters, in family therapy it may not be clear as to who the patient is. The symptomatic family member is often thought by the family to be the patient, but the family therapist may designate the whole family system as the patient or as involved persons in the treatment. The family therapist must be aware of the ethical issues implied in involving the family in the treatment process, and in considering their contribution to the problem and the solution, when they did not originally see themselves as such and did not explicitly contract for treatment.

Because family therapy often involves meeting with all or most of the family members, the family therapist may be in the position of asking certain nonsymptomatic individuals to attend sessions against their wishes. This may involve urging resistant adults and minors both to attend. This situation may become particularly troublesome if a previously nonsymptomatic individual comes to family therapy and becomes distressed.

At times it may be difficult to decide whether a therapeutic action or suggestion may be helpful for one individual, but not helpful or even temporarily harmful to another individual. In their concern for the healthy functioning of the system as a whole, therapists may inadvertently ignore what is best for one individual. An ethical issue is how the decision is made. Should it be the therapist's concern alone, or should it be shared with the family? How much information should they be given on the pros and cons of modalities? Our bias is to negotiate and give the family all the relevant information so that they can make the most informed decision possible.

Secrets and Confidentiality

Unless a therapist sees all the members of a family together at all times, he or she will eventually face a situation in which family secrets are disclosed in individual sessions. Because secrets are a common source of family dysfunction, discovering and dealing with them is a frequent occurrence. As Imber-Black (1993) has stated:

> secrets, decisions about secrecy and openness, and the management of information are woven into the fabric of our society. The paradoxes of what is to be kept secret and what is to be shared and with whom are all around us and are embedded in each encounter between family and therapist. (p. 15)

The family therapist needs to make a distinction between secrecy and privacy. The term *privacy* is usually considered to mean information held by one person that he or she would prefer not to share but that does not directly affect his or her relationship with others. It usually implies a zone of comfort that is free from intrusion. *Secrets* are usually considered to be feelings or information that would directly affect a relationship. They are most often connected to fear, anxiety, and shame, and are often shared—that is, some people in the system know, whereas some do not. There is also a gray area in which different people have different ideas about whether the information is important. (For example, is an affair that occurred during the marriage but ended 10 years ago private or secret?)

Secrets define hierarchy and relationship, leaving the unaware individuals mystified and out of alliance. Some secrets are helpful in that they promote differentiation and separation in less powerful members of a group (e.g., a 6-year-old who says to his sister, "Don't tell Mom we ate the cookies," is learning that parents cannot read the children's minds and that they have some autonomy). Some secrets are dangerous in that proper action will not be taken by the unaware (e.g., an adolescent who says to his sister, "Don't tell Mom we were drinking and driving without a license," leaves parents unable to keep the children safe). Some secrets are about the past, such as an affair many years ago, and some are about the present, such as an ongoing affair or an impending bankruptcy. Most toxic secrets are in some way related to sex (including abortion and illegitimate birth), money, or betrayal.

In general, the best rule of thumb is that a secret should be disclosed if it is seriously affecting the connections between people, poses danger to a family member (e.g., sexual abuse), or shapes family coalitions and alliances. In general, keeping secrets is such a serious barrier that it is better to disclose them, even if painful, because otherwise the sense of mystification and isolation in the unaware is very strong. This principle seems to be true in many areas that affect children and that were formerly always kept secret, such as adoption, out-of-wedlock birth, and artificial insemination. Such issues are, however, very dependent on situation. For example, if adult children choose not to disclose their homosexuality to their parents, this should be considered private, because adults' sexuality is considered to be their own concern. (Because such a secret maintains a significant barrier between children and parents, however, the children should in most cases be encouraged to tell.) However, if a husband is bisexual or homosexual and does not tell his wife but engages in unprotected (or even protected) intercourse with men, the wife is in serious danger and needs to know. Because the husband's sexuality is definitely the wife's concern, not telling her this secret is a serious threat to the relationship.

The therapist must carefully consider the timing and type of disclosure. Premature disclosure before the therapist has formed an alliance with the family can cause the family to leave therapy with no place to deal with potentially explosive material. This is particularly true when there has been a history of violence or abuse. It is generally believed that if the family member refuses to disclose a secret that is so serious that therapy will be derailed, the therapist may terminate therapy but should not disclose the secret. An exception is in cases of potential violence to another, especially in child abuse or homicidal threats, in which the therapist is required to report to the authorities and the potential victim; in such cases the secret must be disclosed. Many therapists feel confused about the requirement to report, knowing that this disclosure may end their relationship with the family. This confusion is difficult to manage, and these cases must be discussed with a supervisor or mentor. Issues concerning disclosure also arise in cases where one partner is HIV positive and has not disclosed this to the other partner. Legally, the therapist is not obliged to do disclose this information—ethically, however, it is extraordinarily difficult not to do so. The patient should be strongly urged to disclose such a secret.

The therapist who works with families in which there are multiple caregiving systems—school, welfare, social services—is constantly faced with decisions about what to share with other caregivers and with the public record. If family members have individual therapists in addition to the therapist for family work, they may or may not want the family therapist to talk with these other therapists. It is strongly recommended that connections be established among all therapists who are involved with a family in order to keep split and mixed agendas from complicating treatment.

Confidentiality issues arise with family members outside the family as it is defined in the treatment group. For example, what information can be given to a concerned grandmother about a child who might be abused? What is owed to the noncustodial parent if the custodial parent and children have been the family of treatment? The therapist must help the family to consider what is in their best interest. In general, interested parties are better brought into the therapy room as potential allies than ignored. However, the need to maintain boundaries between the nuclear family and other family members must also be carefully considered. In general, any disclosures should be discussed at length with the family.

■ ETHICS IN A MANAGED CARE WORLD

Confidentiality is difficult to keep when a managed care expert must give permission for increased sessions, hospitalization, and so forth. Each therapist must consider his or her own willingness to accept the rules of a given managed care company and to fight for patients' and families' right to adequate treatment.

Accordingly, we advise family therapists to take a proactive stance on the basis of the principles elucidated earlier. The therapist first formulates a careful diagnosis of the relevant issues of not only the patient but also the family. Second, the therapist lays out a treatment plan based on models of intervention presented here. Third, the case is presented to the new "member of the treatment team"— a managed care supervisor.

■ INFORMED CONSENT

Our bias is to inform the family of possible difficulties that may arise with therapy, such as poor outcomes or temporary exacerbation of symptoms during treatment. If the therapist believes that problems may occur, as with a patient with an Axis I disorder, it seems quite appropriate and even necessary for the therapist to clearly state and negotiate the treatment goals with the family so that they can make an informed judgment about their desire to embark on the therapy. This negotiation should take place both at the onset and throughout the therapy. If during the evaluation the therapist discerns family secrets to be central to the family problem, he or she may want to inform the family that those issues may need to be a focus of therapy.

More importantly, we agree with Gutheil et al. (1984) that the sharing of uncertainty through the informed consent procedure can be a focal point in building a therapeutic alliance. Those authors point out that "[i]ncreasingly, patients and families who experience tragic disappointment in their expectations…attempt to assuage their grief, helplessness, and despair by blaming…the physicians" (p. 49). This sharing can be done by understanding the origins of the fantasies of certainty, empathizing with unrealistic wishes, and weaning the family from the fantasy of certainty.

■ FINANCIAL ISSUES

Who pays the bill is a relatively simple question in individual treatment with adult patients, but in marital and family work the issue is more complicated. The ethical issues of who pays the bill become especially tense in marital treatment of spouses in conflict. For example, if both spouses have insurance coverage from their respective employers, whose insurance should be used? This question becomes most delicate when the spouses have conflicting views of the matter for any number of reasons, such as not wanting a secretary or co-worker to see insurance forms or not wanting to be identified as a patient. As with many concrete issues of conflict, the family therapist should approach the matter with a sense of fairness. The symbolic meanings of who pays should be thoroughly explored. When the partners have separate incomes and separate financial arrangements, they should each pay half of the bill. Divorced couples may negotiate bitterly over who pays bills for family sessions. If a family session is held between adults and their parents, the question of who pays must be discussed with great care. Most often the person or persons requesting the session pays for it.

Other financial questions involve sudden changes of fortune. For example, if a woman who is married to a well-to-do man divorces and her income drops severely and suddenly, the therapist must address the question of whether to continue treatment even if the husband refuses to pay.

For many therapists and clients, money is the most taboo subject, even more so than sex. It is the therapist's job to clarify his or her own understanding and feelings about money in order to be able to support discussions with patients.

■ PROFESSIONAL ISSUES

Boundaries and Dual Relationships

The issue of boundaries and dual relationships is a critical one in all forms of psychotherapy. Because couples and family therapy involves more than one patient in the consulting room, there is less likelihood of inappropriate sexual contact between therapist and patient. However, there have been cases in which a therapist, working with a couple, began an affair with one of the spouses, either during couples therapy or after the couple separated. Therapists may also have other forms of dual relationships. For example, a therapist may agree to treat the child of a colleague. This makes a very confusing boundary for the child, who may wonder what the therapist will tell the parent. In such cases the therapist will have a very difficult time remaining neutral if family sessions are needed. Therapists who treat students or supervisees directly under them in training programs are also engaging in behavior considered to be unethical, because the vulnerability of the patient puts him or her at a serious disadvantage as a student who must be graded or evaluated.

Other confusing questions may arise because the issues that families face are the same as those faced by therapists in their personal lives, making it very likely that at some point countertransference issues will become ethical ones. For example, seeing a couple going through a separation at the same time that one is going through the early stages of one's own divorce is an extremely difficult thing to do, and the likelihood of remaining neutral to both parties is not great. Although it is obviously impossible for a therapist to stop treating patients while going through a divorce, he or she could certainly choose not to accept a new couple or family whose situation is very similar to his or her own.

Coding and Billing

Family therapists often ask how to code for couples therapy. The American Psychiatric Association's Committee on Practice and Managed Care suggests the following. Because there is no Current Procedural Terminology (CPT) code for couples therapy per se, they suggest using CPT code 90847 and designating one of the partners as the patient. This code is used when the therapy includes the patient and family members. CPT code 90846 is family therapy without the patient present. They recommend not billing separately for each party and, if two insurance companies are involved, billing the one with the better reimbursement rate or better coverage.

Medicare does not cover any kind of couples therapy. One of the partners has to be designated as the patient. The Medicare manual states that family psychotherapy services are covered only when the primary purpose is the treatment of the individual patient's condition. The issues revolve around a need to observe and correct the patient's interaction with family members (or caregivers) or in the management of the patient.

Training and Licensure

Professional licensure has been a recent development in the field of marital and family therapy. The Association of Marital and Family Therapy Regulating Boards of the American Association for Marriage and Family Therapy has developed a consensus about a fundamental knowledge base. As a unique profession, the practice of marital and family therapy means "the application of psychotherapeutic and family systems theories and techniques to the delivery of services to individuals, couples, and families in order to diagnose and treat a nervous and mental disorder" (American Association for Marriage and Family Therapy 1991). On the basis of this definition, a national Examination in Marital and Family Therapy now exists. This examination covers the following domains:

- Joining, assessment, and diagnosis
- Designing treatment
- Conducting the course of treatment
- Establishing and maintaining appropriate networks
- Assessing the outcome of treatment
- Maintaining professional standards

As of 2001, 44 states regulate marital and family therapists. There are an estimated 46,000 marital and family therapists in the United States (American Association for Marriage and Family Therapy 2002).

Competencies

To protect the public from untrained, incompetent, and/or unethical family therapists and family intervention, there must be a clear delineation of the competencies needed to conduct family therapy. In addition, ways of teaching and assessing the presence (or absence) of these competencies must be developed. Following are some of the qualities that we think are important for the family therapist, in addition to those required to conduct other therapies.

- Tolerance of family fighting
- Comfortableness with family secrets
- Ability to adapt to different technical models or to mix different schools of therapy together in a treatment package
- Interest in issues of gender, diversity, class, and culture
- Ability to be active and directive

In addition, we have a strong bias that, in the training of family therapists, attention should be paid to the humanistic qualities of integrity, respect, and compassion for patients and their families. Attainment of these qualities is critical to the outcome of therapy. Therapists must come to realize that they are not omnipotent.

For successful long-term outcomes, both family and therapist(s) must play a part. The therapist may, for example, recognize a family's need to be cared for or inability to make decisions, but it is not his or her responsibility to take over in these respects. Rather, the therapeutic task is to help the family to recognize its difficulties and to start seeking solutions. Although therapists may decide to accept responsibility for providing a setting, establishing and maintaining a therapeutic alliance, and offering observations and suggestions, those who take considerably greater responsibility for change are diluting what energy and motivation the family might have, as well as being likely candidates for burnout (Lask 1986).

Finally, the therapist should remember that the everyday practice of family therapy is untidy and disorderly. At times therapists fail and make mistakes (and regret them) (Spellman and Harper 1996).

■ FINAL ISSUES

A final issue is the marginalization of the field. The key implication for the trainee is, as Kramer (1995) has warned, that family therapy as a modality might not be reimbursed (like other forms of psychotherapy) "because it conforms poorly to contemporary models of research." Of course, the field has been working on issues of reimbursement, and trainee and supervisor need to cover this nonreimbursement issue in the course of training so that patients can be treated properly.

Historically, as family therapy developed, differences appeared between the basic assumptions and practices of the field and the tenets of the feminist movement. Early papers challenged the family therapy establishment from a feminist perspective (Hare-Mustin 1978). Inevitably, these issues came under scrutiny in the training and supervision of students. The resulting dialogue has enriched the field and has reshaped the focus of many educational programs. Descriptions of the variety of gender differences have emerged from marital-interaction research, and a rich literature of related training practices has developed (Helmeke 1994; Libow 1985; Nelson 1991; Roberts 1991).

At the end of a family therapy training program, the trainee's education is actually just beginning. In a rapidly changing field such as family therapy, an individual must begin a program of life-long self-education based on a continual awareness of the literature and course work and the need to evaluate his or her own work, to entertain new ideas, and to discard old ones. As obvious as this may seem, it is the inculcation of these principles that identifies the inspired and skillful clinician, teacher, or researcher.

■ REFERENCES

American Association for Marriage and Family Therapy: AAMFT Code of Ethics (2 pp, unpaginated). Washington, DC, American Association for Marriage and Family Therapy, 1991

American Association for Marriage and Family Therapy: Marriage and Family Therapy Licensing & Certification, Directory of State MFT Licensing/Certification Boards, Introduction. Available at http://www.aamft.org/resources/Online_directories/boardcontacts.htm. Accessed June 28, 2002

Boszormenyi-Nagy I, Spark G: Invisible Loyalties: Reciprocity in Intergenerational Family Therapy. New York, Harper and Row, 1973

Gutheil TG, Bursztajn H, Brodsky A: Malpractice prevention through the sharing of uncertainty, informed consent and the therapeutic alliance. N Engl J Med 311:49–51, 1984

Hare-Mustin RT: A feminist approach to family therapy. Fam Proc 17:181–194, 1978

Helmeke KL: Fostering a safe atmosphere: a first step in discussing gender in family therapy training programs. Contemporary Family Therapy 16:503–519, 1994

Imber-Black E: Secrets in families and family therapy. New York, Norton, 1993

Kramer P: Shape of the field. Psychiatric Times, August 1995

Lask B: Whose responsibility. Journal of Family Therapy 8:205–206, 1986

Libow JA: Training family therapists as feminists, in Women and Family Therapy. Edited by Ault-Riche M. Rockville, MD, Aspen, 1985

Nelson TS: Gender in family therapy supervision. Contemporary Family Therapy 13:357–369, 1991

Roberts JM: Sugar and spice, toads and mice: gender issues in family therapy training. Journal of Marital and Family Therapy 17:121–132, 1991

Spellman D, Harper DJ: Failure, mistakes, regret and other subjugated stories in family therapy. Journal of Family Therapy 18:205–214, 1996

INDEX

*Page numbers printed in **boldface** type refer to tables or figures.*